Help for the Hyperactive Child

Help for the
Hyperactive Child

SYDNEY WALKER III, M.D.

HOUGHTON MIFFLIN COMPANY BOSTON

Library of Congress Cataloging in Publication Data

Walker, Sydney.
  Help for the hyperactive child.
  Includes bibliographical references and index.
   1. Hyperactive children. I. Title.
RJ506.H9W35   618.9'28'5884   77-14395
ISBN 0-395-25722-0

Printed in the United States of America

V 10 9 8 7 6 5 4 3

Dedicated to Syd, Sybil, Cleta,
and to a healthier future for all children.

Acknowledgments

The case histories in their full medical details have been taken from the files of patients seen at the Southern California Neuropsychiatric Institute. I have of course altered names and disguised personal details to protect the privacy of the individuals involved. Due to the specialized nature of the neuropsychiatric diagnostic procedures and vocabulary, a major effort went into "translating" this information from its highly technical form into readily understandable language. This was accomplished by the effort of Ronal Kayser, whose tenacious labors and keen understanding of the total picture accomplished the transition from a dry, technical, professional concept to a logical, readable format. I will forever feel grateful to Anita McClellan of the Houghton Mifflin editorial staff for her unstinting efforts and unlimited faith on behalf of *Help for the Hyperactive Child*. The task of preparing a manuscript always requires many helping hands. I was fortunate to have assisting me Jovita Meirick, Judy Kerber, Glenn Klein, Judith Wesling, and Melanie Willis. Emotional support and encouragement throughout the preparation and study were supplied unselfishly by my dear wife, Gail.

Contents

IV. NEUROPSYCHIATRIC DIAGNOSIS: WHAT HOPE IS THERE AHEAD?

PART I
WHAT HYPERACTIVITY IS

1

Childhood's Life-Crippling
Affliction

"I'M SORRY THAT I MUST TELL you this, but as matters stand your child will have to be taken out of our school." The setting could be in any one of many elementary schools in the United States. The speaker may be a teacher, in most cases a preschool, first-grade, or second-grade teacher. Or the message may be delivered by the school's principal. In either case, the voice and manner are quietly sympathetic and very firmly authoritative.

The listener is the child's parent, sometimes both parents, but usually the mother. Quite possibly this has been you or your spouse. Or, if your child is not yet in school, your turn may come next year or in the years ahead. The chances of that happening will be greater if your youngster is a boy, since in four out of five (sometimes in nine out of ten) cases, as they are detected in the schools, the affected child is of the male sex.

The teacher or principal continues: "Billy simply isn't achieving anything here. He's unable to do the work, and can't keep up with the rest of the class. And it's not fair to the other thirty children because he's such a disruptive influence in the school-room."

Then, Billy's parent may be shown a mimeographed Behavior and Learning Rating Scale, which bears Billy's name and itemizes such conduct as:

Sits fiddling with small objects
Hums and makes other odd noises

Is restless or overactive
Easily excitable, temper outbursts
Overly sensitive
Makes excessive demands for teacher's attention
Teases other children, disrupts activities

The rating scale includes such other educational shortcomings as:

Erratic learning behavior
Difficulty in reading
Difficulty in writing
Difficulty in calculations
Difficulty in memory
Short attention span
Seldom completes assignments
Does not follow directions

It also lists the child's motor activity problems:

Appears awkward, clumsy, with abnormal gait
Handwriting poor
Speech sounds are inaccurate or immature

The mother protests. "I realize that Billy is more high-strung than most kids. He's nervous and flighty, and not the brightest child in the world. But he's not so stupid he can't learn! That I refuse to believe."

The school's representative does not disagree. "Oh, I haven't said that Billy is stupid. He's probably up to the average in intelligence or better than average. It's his behavior that keeps him from learning. He's forever whispering, jumping up, talking out of turn, starting quarrels, even getting into fights. And there's no use trying to discipline or punish him, for Billy can't help what he's doing. He is what we call a hyperactive child with minimal brain dysfunction."

Billy's mother sits silently. Like many of the parents observed by Dr. Paul H. Wender, professor of psychiatry at the University of Idaho's College of Medicine, she is aware that her son has a history of hyperactive disturbance reaching back to his second year of life, and perhaps farther. Dr. Wender has stated that half of all hyperactive youngsters are identified as such in the first grade, at five or six years of age. The remaining half are described by their parents as having always been "peculiar," or different from their brothers and sisters, some even having been recognized as hyperactive before and from birth.[1]

Billy's mother has been spared the anguish described by a young woman who brought her four-month-old baby into Dr. T. Berry Brazelton's office. "I get so desperate that I want to smother him or put him so far away I can't hear him. I'm afraid I might drop him or hurt him. I can't stand this baby." The woman's graphic description makes one wonder how much child abuse may be associated with hyperactivity in very young children.[2]

Billy's parent cannot deny that her child as an infant was "a squirmer, never a cuddler," and that as he grew older he was "a handful" at home, always "up to something" and "into things," accident-prone, forgetful, quick-tempered — the kind of child who makes a parent eager to leave the home early in the morning and stay late at the office; the kind of child who prods an overwrought parent into longing for the day when he can be sent off to school. And then this!

"But — keep him at home? What then? What are we supposed to do?" Her head is a clutter of half-snatched-at, then hastily rejected possibilities. Hire a tutor? Send Billy to an expensive private school? Even perhaps place him in a state institution for the feeble-minded? . . . It is too horrible to contemplate. But she has to consider, too, what will be fair to Billy's brothers and sisters.

"Well. Of course that's not what I said," the teacher or principal corrects. "What I told you was, 'as matters stand.' Actually, all over the country thousands of children who have Billy's condition are able to remain in school and do well in their studies — when they are given the proper medication. Of course, it's for you to decide, but I certainly suggest that you talk with your family doctor about a prescription to help Billy behave normally."

"Oh?" A hesitant pause. "Then, this . . . brain damage is curable?"

Another correction. "Not damage exactly. Brain dysfunction. So I wouldn't say cure exactly. But often the symptoms can be brought under control, and eventually — that is, six or seven years from now — Billy should outgrow his condition."

Billy's hyperactive "condition," or "disorder," is not merely an excess of the normal youthful exuberance, enthusiasm, and high spirits that characterize the play of healthy, vigorous children. The hyperactive child is overactive in pointless, restless, distractive, uncontrollable, fidgety, impulsive, demanding, destructive, impatient, often hostile, quarrelsome, intolerant, defiant, and unhappy ways. The hyperactive youngster may seem unable to wait his or her turn in games, or being served at the table, and if denied immediate gratification may explode into a tantrum or burst into sobs of frustration. Such a child is often unable to make friends with other children, and is instead disliked and rejected. Yet other hyperactive children are fearful, shrinking, withdrawn, and prone to fits of sobbing. Also, not infrequently, hyperactivity occurs in modified degrees and may sometimes be recognized and identified only after careful scrutiny by a properly trained professional observer.

In each child's case, we must first be sure that hyperactivity exists. It may not, despite the findings recorded on an educational rating scale. The clues that point, or seem to point, to hyperactivity and minimal brain dysfunction are *behavioral* clues. As such they are not objective, identifiable, and measurable — as, for instance, are cholesterol and triglycerides in a laboratory blood sampling. In the schoolroom and on the playground, teachers and supervisors observe that certain children are "overactive," "hard to manage," "explosive and aimless" in what they do, "uncooperative" in what they are asked to do, "silly," "immature," "sassy," and are "unpopular" with their classmates and with themselves ("have poor self-images"), and are "aggressive" or "exhibit precocious sexual interests."

At what point on the scale of human behavior does the healthy activity of childhood become unhealthy overactivity? How hard is "hard to manage," and for whom is it hard? Evaluations of this kind are akin to the judgments that "Rob is a real live wire, up and at 'em boy," while "Jeff is just a roughneck," and "Jim is a sissy," and that "Alice is such a sweet, ladylike little girl," but "Elsie's a tomboy." Such determinations are subjective. They involve not only the behavior of the child under inspection, but also the attitudes of the adult observers as well as the social environment in which the persons involved live and to which they react. Sociological and economic factors influence behavior of children who grow up surrounded by alcoholism, drug addiction, shoplifting, quarreling, hysterics, desertion, child neglect, abuse, molestation, and by juvenile delinquency. Family attitudes matter. An older sibling's gibe, "School is a bummer. You'll hate it," can be a self-fulfilling prophecy.

It may seem paradoxical, but in medical fact a child's behavior may provide no sure indication of the severity of the youngster's hyperactivity problem. Medically viewed, the hyperactivity disorder is seen as a syndrome, a constellation of signs and symptoms that collectively indicate the abnormal condition. To say that these children are hyperactive is not at all the same thing as declaring that all of them have some *one* more or less obscure but specific ailment. Nor is it to imply that the syndrome can be controlled or suppressed by means of psychoactive drugs. Least of all is it the same thing as saying that as the hyperactive child grows older his or her ailment will be outgrown.

All that we can state, on the evidence provided by the young patient's behavior and school achievement, is that this child exhibits a visible hyperactivity that is not in itself a disease, but that indicates an existing disorder, in somewhat the same way that coughing or dizziness or headaches (which, by the way, frequently occur in the hyperactivity syndrome) are not in themselves diseases, but symptoms of illness. HYPERACTIVITY IS ITSELF A SYMPTOM AND INDICATES THAT AN UNDIAGNOSED SOMETHING, SOMEWHERE IN THE CHILD'S MAKE-UP, IS AMISS — ORGANICALLY AMISS OR FUNCTIONALLY AMISS.

Let us reconsider the suggestion that little Billy should be given a prescription drug to stabilize his hyperactive behavior.

Clearly, a diagnosis of minimal brain dysfunction — or any diagnosis that has the effect of declaring a child's health problem to be exclusively *malfunctional* in its origin or in its nature — cannot safely be made until a reasonable effort has first been devoted to exploring the possibility of an organic defect existing either as the source of the child's problem or allied with it. Therefore, numerous physiological defects and various toxicities that are common in our modern life must be ruled out through testing procedures. Diagnosis that will provide the guidelines for truly effective treatment must be differential; it must isolate and identify *every* cause that contributes to a child's hyperactive behavior and learning disabilities or dysfunctions. (For example, is Billy one of the many small children whose hyperactivity is caused by chronic lead poisoning? See Chapter 19 for a complete description of a differential diagnosis.)

Billy's behavior and poor school achievement suggest a central nervous system disorder. The central nervous system guides the human being's sitting, standing, walking, and talking, eating and drinking, and all other voluntary actions. Through its component autonomic nervous system, it regulates the activities of all the bodily mechanisms, organs, and glands. It is responsive to both physical and emotional needs. The eyes tear when a grain of dust touches an eyeball and when a person is stricken with grief. Sometimes the mouth waters at the prospect of food; at another time it may dry and the throat muscles refuse to swallow. In shock or in illness, the stomach may eject its contents: vomiting is a common symptom in children's illnesses, and projectile vomiting has its own special significance. Spasms, including involuntary facial grimaces or tics, are another expression of central nervous system activity.

Hyperactivity is central nervous system malactivity. In many children, the symptoms can be modified or relieved temporarily by a stimulant drug. But the respite lasts only a few hours, and the drug poses many recognized perils. Such medication ignores the truly significant problem to be explored. Why, in each individual child's case, does the central nervous system malfunction?

Why is Billy awkward, with abnormal gait? Why his stammering speech and blinking eyes? Why does he fidget, hum, demand attention, burst into sobs? Why has he so little self-control? Is there something physically wrong, organically wrong? This kind of preliminary research is necessary even in cases where an emotional pathology has been identified as unresolved Oedipal complex, pathological parent-child relationship, or antisocial behavior. The child's biological integrity is nevertheless important. The resolution of the emotional pathology will be much more readily and firmly achieved if the patient does not have a contributing metabolic, toxic, or infectious process going on at the same time.

It seems totally obvious that the hyperactive child's biological status should be explored *before* he or she is put on a regimen of drug treatment that cannot cure, but will mask, the symptoms of his or her disorder. Clearly, the family doctor cannot be expected to go beyond the scope of a general physical examination to undertake the complete neurological evaluation that is required to search out and interpret the hard but hidden medical evidence.

Nor is the task one that the elementary school teacher is qualified to take in hand. This is not to disparage the load that classroom teachers have borne in their contacts with these highly difficult children day after day, year in and year out. For teachers and children alike, the school experience can be energy-draining, morale-challenging, nerve-racking, and heartbreaking. The enforced physical inaction, disciplined quiet, concentration, and attention to the lesson material are painful for hyperactive youngsters. Such burdensome conditions put a severe strain upon an adult trying to relate to children who even in the favorable circumstances of their recreational play are unable to keep their attention focused on activities of their own choice. Teachers, many of whom hold M.A.'s in their field, must feel reduced to baby-sitter status when their efforts, no matter how dedicated, are rewarded by scanty success or no success at all. Yet, unhappily, learning disability means

exactly this: The child who is unable to learn is unteachable —
or, at least, cannot be taught by the usual group methods in the
usual schoolroom setting.

Educators' professional journals have generally demonstrated
candor and common sense in their reporting and recommendations on hyperactivity. These publications reflect a growing
concern with the *magnitude* of the incidence of hyperactivity
among schoolchildren, reckoned in 1971 as 3 out of 100 elementary school youngsters[3] — an estimate that by 1974 had been replaced by others, ranging as high as 10 per cent[4] of all grade
school children. The top 1974 estimate reached an astonishingly
high figure, and yet one that pales in comparison with the 40 per
cent cited by two critics of the schools' role in coping with the
problem.[5] The 40 per cent estimate, however, appears to have
been arrived at by combining estimates of "learning disabilities"
with estimates of "hyperkinesis."*

In practical fact, almost all children classified as hyperactive by
the schools have severe learning handicaps, and almost all who
are considered to have minimal brain dysfunction or learning
disabilities are seen as being hyperactive. Questions may arise as
to when the hyperactive condition is "primary," with the learning disability "secondary" to it, or vice versa; and it has been acknowledged in the educational periodicals that as a term
"hyperactivity" "is imprecise and covers a multitude of characteristics and behaviors."[6]

In practice, the steps that have actually been taken with the
hyperactive child, and that are still being taken today, are determined by what is available and feasible in each child's school,
community, and immediate family situation. A few children — a
very small minority — are examined by specially qualified diagnosticians. Some others are treated as disciplinary problems.
Many — no one knows exactly how many — are being "medi-

*Educators tend to employ such terms as "hyperactive syndrome," "learning
disability," and "specific learning disability." The medical profession inclines toward "hyperkinetic syndrome" and "minimal brain dysfunction (MBD)." The
meanings are much the same: The child is behaviorally hyperactive and educationally handicapped.

cated" with one or the other of two stimulant drugs, Ritalin or
Dexedrine. No nationwide statistics are available, but from local
figures Dr. Mark A. Stewart of the University of Iowa extrapo-
lated a "ball park estimate" of 800,000 children for whom these
drugs were being prescribed in early 1976.[7]

The only acceptable defense for the widespread drugging of
young children today would be that tentatively phrased by
Joseph N. Murray, professor of school psychology at Kent University. Among possible causes of hyperkinesis, wrote Professor
Murray, "the delayed maturation concept is considered important by many, since it suggests that a youngster can 'outgrow' his
hyperkinetic problem. If this is valid, then hyperkinesis must
necessarily be controlled by medication so that the youngster
won't miss out on the basics of learning important in later life."[8]

Evidence is now accumulating that hyperactivity is not outgrown in any meaningful sense. The hyperactive behavior may
lessen somewhat, but the underlying causes breed other and
more serious symptoms. Such is the appraisal reached by
Dorothea M. Ross, research psychologist at the University of
California Medical School, San Francisco, and Sheila A. Ross,
senior research associate at the Palo Alto Medical Research
Foundation. The Rosses find evidence that adolescence is an
even more difficult life phase for the hyperactive child than are
the years of middle childhood. To accept a lessening of activity
as a positive prognosis for the hyperactive child, they say, is to
oversimplify the problem grossly. The Rosses cite in detail from
various studies, all of which indicate that many formerly
hyperactive children continue to have difficulties in adolescence, including school problems, unsatisfactory family and peer
relations, and trouble with the law. As the Rosses evaluate the
evidence, hyperactivity does not vanish in adolescence. It di-
minishes, but the adolescent is still noticeably more restless, distractive, impulsive, and less stable emotionally than others of his
or her age. They cite underachievement, attentional difficulties,
poor self-esteem, and depression as major problems.[9]

True, as late as 1975, Dr. J. Gordon Millichap, of the depart-

ments of neurology and pediatrics at Northwestern University
Medical School, in his "questions and answers" discussion of this
subject asked whether parents could expect a lessening of their
children's hyperactivity with increasing age. He stated that it was
usual for behavior to become more controlled and goal-directed
as children reach puberty. He postulated a delayed development
of the brain to explain some minimal brain dysfunction syn-
dromes. In concluding his answer, he said that the use of medication such as Ritalin is often unnecessary after twelve or fourteen years of age.[10]

But Dr. Millichap, who was once the bellwether in his field,
does not tell concerned parents how much more control is
"more," or how many are "some." The reader who wants to
know what is in store for his or her child, or for the children in
his or her classroom, will find the Millichap statement vitiated by
its vagueness.

Quite a different conclusion was reached in 1976 by Dr. Dennis P. Cantwell, of UCLA's Neuropsychiatric Institute. He
criticizes as "unjustified" the optimism of the early investigators,
who tended to emphasize their view that the hyperactive child
syndrome was a time-limited condition that disappeared naturally as the patient grew older. The *symptom*, so Dr. Cantwell
stresses, may diminish with age, but not so the eventual outcome.
Cantwell devotes twelve pages to discussing recent studies of the
outcome in the adolescent years and later lives of hyperactive
children. In summarizing the findings, Cantwell states that as
these children mature they are prone to develop significant
psychiatric and social problems. They have been found especially liable to antisocial behavior, serious academic retardation,
and depression. As adults, their likely conditions appear to be
alcoholism, hysteria, and perhaps psychosis. Cantwell further
reports that the studies do not clearly demonstrate that treatment of any type significantly affects the long-term outcome for
the hyperactive child.[11] (The studies discussed by Dr. Cantwell
do not refer to neuropsychiatric diagnosis and the outcomes resulting from its use. There has never been a study of the kind of
diagnosis described in this book.)

One of the first published investigations of adolescent hyperactivity is that made by Dr. Wallace Mendelson, Dr. Noel Johnson, and Dr. Mark A. Stewart. The three psychiatrists collected the names of 140 children who had been observed either in the Psychiatry Clinic of the St. Louis Children's Hospital or in Dr. Stewart's practice. These were children who had been diagnosed by psychiatrists as having the hyperactivity syndrome. At the time of the subsequent investigation, they had reached the stage of puberty, at which time it has been supposed that the syndrome would have been outgrown.

This study of adolescents with earlier histories of overactivity syndrome found that "about half of the children were markedly improved, one quarter remained unchanged and the remaining quarter lay in between." In its admirably presented details, the Mendelson, Johnson, and Stewart report says much more — and much less — than can be read into its quoted, summarizing statement. At follow-up, more than half of the adolescents in the study were still receiving psychiatric assistance — a circumstance that does nothing to support a theory of spontaneously waning and disappearing hyperactivity.

Indeed, the report asserted that "most of the children were still having trouble with the major symptoms . . . though the intensity of the symptoms had often improved. Three out of four children were giving their parents a great deal of trouble because they would not obey rules in the home; many of the children were moody and suffered from a lack of self-esteem and a chip on the shoulder." Also, "one measure of how the parents felt about these children was that two out of five had seriously considered sending their child away to a military school or Boys Town, and half (46 per cent) were unable to think of a career for which their child was suited."[12]

The antisocial behavior that Mendelson, Johnson, and Stewart found in many of the 83 twelve-to-sixteen-year-old youths is typically seen in youngsters with learning disability. Professor Allan Berman, a University of Rhode Island psychologist, has stated that between 70 and 90 per cent of juvenile delinquents countrywide have a learning problem. Berman told a national conference on the subject that parents, educators, and law enforcement officers have failed to cope with juvenile delinquency because they have failed to perceive its link to learning disabilities. He indicated that arrests of youths climbed 140 per cent between 1968 and 1977 compared with a 20 per cent rise for offenders over eighteen years of age, and he cited a 250 per cent rise in violent youth crimes, twice that of adults during the same years.[13]

How much can existing, drug-oriented remedial programs claim to be accomplishing for these children? How much better off are the youngsters for having spent years on alleviative medication? It is by no means safe to rely on the unproved proposition that children will "outgrow" disorders affecting their behavior and learning ability. It is even probable that no child ever outgrows the hyperactive syndrome — except the ones who succeed in throwing off the effects of an undiagnosed underlying deficiency or disorder.

The problem is serious. The problem is national. We are told that hundreds of thousands of our country's young children are engulfed in a mind- and life-destroying catastrophe. TRAGICALLY, OUR EDUCATIONAL, MEDICAL, AND PHARMACEUTICAL ESTABLISHMENTS HAVE COME UP WITH NOTHING BEYOND A HEAD IN THE SAND, SELF-BLINDING STRATEGY OF TREATING THE SYMPTOMS INSTEAD OF SEEKING TO IDENTIFY AND CURE THE UNDERLYING CAUSES.

2

A History of Hyperactivity

THE RECORD OF HYPERACTIVITY in children is recent and brief. The disorder's first appearance in medical literature occurred in 1902 in the *Lancet*, which published lectures on the subject by an English pediatrician, Dr. G. F. Still. However, hyperactive behavior had been observed in individual children before then. Dorothea M. Ross and Sheila A. Ross dedicated their scholarly work *Hyperactivity: Research-Theory-Action* to "a real stalwart whose warmth, wisdom, and steadfast refusal to accept the school's negative appraisals as final gave a very hyperactive child the support he needed in his troubled years." The stalwart was an English nanny; the very hyperactive child was Winston Churchill, who was born in 1876. A number of writers have alluded to the hyperactive childhood of Thomas Alva Edison, who was born in 1847, thought ineducable in school, and who was taught at home by his remarkable mother. There are other nationally and internationally famous examples.

Hyperactivity as a recognized syndrome is a recent development. As a fact of life, it has pretty surely been around for many centuries, during which its symptoms were usually considered evidence of poor moral character or of stupidity. Possibly "witches" were hanged for casting spells on such children.

Certainly in the United States, through the nation's first century and well into its second, social and economic conditions tended to draw a veil over the presence of whatever hyperactivity existed. Disparate, disadvantaged individuals stand out most visibly when placed in otherwise homogeneous groups, and are most obviously inadequate in competitive situations. The population of "melting pot" America was extremely heterogeneous. During the years from 1820 to 1930, three out of five of the world's immigrants landed on American shores. These immigrants were for the most part young adults. Any difficulties an immigrant's child had in school could be attributed to the foreign language and Old Country ways in the youngster's home background.

At least half of the hyperactivity noted among today's children is first identified in the classroom. The school environment is highly competitive. Every minute of the school day children are being observed and classified in terms of reading, writing, arithmetic, spelling, hygiene, citizenship, punctuality, creativity, or good citizenship on the playground. In our pioneer past, until the 1850s, no state in the Union had compulsory education. In the slaveholding states, there were often laws prohibiting the education of black children.

Who needed much education to earn a living then? Typewriters had not been invented, Florence Nightingale had not made nursing a respectable profession, and the teachers of the period were schoolmasters. Almost the only "profession" open to women was that of hired girl. For males who did not make it through school, the growing country had a large and lively demand for cowboys and muleskinners, pick and shovel miners and ditchdiggers, gandydancers to lay railroad tracks, loggers to fell forests with handaxes and two-man saws, and for pickers of cotton and corn. None of these jobs required book learning. Rural America remained in the hand- and horse-powered stage of agriculture through the first third of the twentieth century, and there is still some lingering dependence upon "stoop labor."

During most of our national history, Americans have prized (or have professed to prize) the virtues of ambition, hard work, stick-to-itiveness, and the ant-versus-grasshopper morality. It is not an attitude that lends itself to a sympathetic understanding of a young flibbertigibbet. If we like, we may speculate how much hyperactive disorder existed in our past, how often it was viewed as a moral flaw in the child, and how often its pathophysiological symptoms were treated with old-fashioned herbal recipes for "nervousness," "nervous irritation," "sleeplessness," "nervous twitching," "tremors," and "restlessness."

In part, we may attribute the twentieth century's quickened awareness of hyperactivity to two separate but almost simultaneous developments. The first was educational.

In 1905, Alfred Binet and Theodore Simon devised an intelligence test that was used to identify retarded children in the schools of France. In recent years we have come to take a sophisticated, skeptical attitude toward intelligence testing, and we question what value to attach to such tests. Intelligence testing in our pluralistic society can indeed be challenged as a faulty, not truly objective measurement of a disadvantaged, minority group individual's capacities. Even so, it seems more objective than the personal observations and judgments of individual teachers, supervisors, principals, and district superintendents. It is often said that the only value I.Q. really measures is what it takes to get along in school. Even if that were all the Simon-Binet and its successor tests ever proved, it would be enough to indicate that what causes most hyperactive children's school failures is *not* stupidity. Modern tests show that these children are in the normal range of intelligence, even when intelligence is narrowly defined as educability.

Also across the Atlantic, in 1906, Sigmund Freud began his milestone efforts with Jung, Adler, and others. The new science of psychiatry was on its way. Again, in recent years we have come to take a more sophisticated, skeptical view of much in Freud's teaching. Nevertheless, psychiatry and its associated fields of study — psychotherapy, psychoanalysis, psychosomatic medicine, and psychopharmacology — have defined an area in which emotional disturbances manifest themselves in the guise of physical disorders. Some of these manifestations are further defined as affecting organs of the body that are governed by the autonomic function of the central nervous system, thus setting psychosomatic illness apart from hysteria, which Freud in his early studies characterized as affecting the portions of the body that are under voluntary control.

The links connecting Dr. Still's hyperactivity, Binet-Simon's test, and Freud's psychiatry were not apparent in the early 1900s. Three decades passed before a fourth significant element appeared. The period was the Great Depression decade. The scene was the Emma Pendleton Bradley Home at East Providence, Rhode Island, an institution for resident patients of normal intelligence, most of them children under twelve years of age with neurological and behavioral disorders. The home had its own hospital, school, and recreational facilities. The children were closely watched, and records of their behavior were made as part of the everyday routine. Dr. Charles Bradley, the institution's director, believed that the young patients were quite unaware of this continuous surveillance.

Dr. Bradley was well acquainted with the studies being made of Benzedrine (the registered trademark of amphetamine sulfate, an amphetamine product at that time new), studies in which the drug's effects upon adults were being investigated and reported in the medical journals. Nothing had been published on how children would react to Benzedrine. Would some of the changes noted in adult patients be of value in treating children with behavioral problems? To find out, Dr. Bradley planned an experiment.

The children were already being watched routinely and their behavior recorded by ward nurses and teachers. During the week-long trial with Benzedrine, and for the weeks preceding and following the test, a special psychiatric nurse carefully observed each child.

While they were receiving daily morning doses of Benzedrine, 14 of the 30 children were reported as showing "a great increase of interest in school material . . . Speed of comprehension and accuracy of performance were increased in most cases . . . The improvement was noted in all school subjects. It appeared promptly the first day Benzedrine was given and disappeared on the first day it was discontinued."[1]

Eight children showed fewer but some changes for the better. One child was under school age. These proportions — a half improved, a quarter somewhat improved, and a quarter unchanged or worsened — reappear in later studies of the effects of amphetamine and amphetamine-type medication. Also recurring is the report of the improvement vanishing when the medication is stopped. In the Bradley study, most of the children's emotional responses, and other psychological and physiological effects, were rather vaguely defined. This might be expected in a testing situation that lasted only one week, during which "questioning the children in regard to their subjective feelings was studiously avoided."

In his published report, Bradley emphasized two aspects of his experiment. The first was: "To see a single daily dose of Benzedrine produce a greater improvement in school performance than the combined efforts of a capable staff working in a most favorable setting would have been all but demoralizing to the teachers, had not the improvement been so gratifying from a practical standpoint."[2] The gratification, however, may have been naive.*

When one reads in Mark A. Stewart and Sally Wendkos Olds's account of the Bradley study, "The children themselves called the medicine 'arithmetic pills,' because they felt they could do their arithmetic more easily when they were taking the drug," it

---

*From the even more practical standpoint of a study in which three groups of hyperactive children were compared by various measures of outcome five years after initial evaluation, an amphetamine-type medication (Ritalin) did not significantly affect their school achievement. The drug was found helpful in making hyperactive children more manageable at home and at school. So reported Dr. Gabrielle Weiss, Ela Kruger, M.S.W., Dr. Ursel Danielson, and Meryl Elman, B.A., on the basis of comparisons of one group of 24 children who were treated with Ritalin for three to five years after an initial evaluation, a second group of 22 treated with chlorpromazine for eighteen months to five years, and a third group who had received no medication during the follow-up period. See also pages 91–92 of this book. *CMA Journal*, January 25, 1975, pp. 159–165.

becomes evident that the children's knowledge of what was going on may have led to self-fulfilling expectations. Dr. Bradley's experiment lacked scrupulous procedures to ensure that neither the patient nor the persons dispensing the medication knew whether a drug or a placebo was being administered.

Bradley's report emphasized the behavior-calming effect of Benzedrine. But how could a stimulant drug "subdue" an aggressive, hyperactive child and yet stimulate a seclusive child to show more initiative and become more active? "It seems paradoxical," he wrote, and evidently the paradox bothered him.* It is unlikely that he was troubled by reflecting that Samuel Hahnemann, more than a century earlier, had founded homeopathic medicine on the theory that "like should be cured by like." Nor could Bradley have foreseen that advocates of stimulant drugs for hyperactive children would in the future cite the "paradoxical effect" in assuming that these children must be physiologically different from most people in ways that make stimulant drug therapy appropriate for them.[4]

As a psychiatrist, he went on working with this enigma through the 1940s. He searched for the origin of children's behavioral problems in the development of emotional conflicts, in the impairment of the child's capacity to deal with his or her conflicts, and in both. He saw the expression of the problem as varying and often appearing to be related more directly to the personality characteristics of each child than to the circumstances that caused the behavior to change. "Certain of these patients uniformly and characteristically showed aggressive, assaultive, hyperkinetic behavior disorders. Others, at the opposite end of the behavior scale, appeared pathologically shy, with-

---

*A drug's action may depend upon the reception it receives in the drug user's body. Alcohol is a common depressant drug whose pick-me-up effect is not paradoxical. A teen-ager's first acquaintance with martinis will induce intoxication very rapidly, for the youth's body doesn't know how to handle the drug. A more seasoned drinker can rapidly consume several martinis without apparent effect; his liver has learned to mass-produce the enzymes to turn the drug into sugars. With an old toper, the outcome may be his death; his liver can no longer stand the gaff. The alcohol in the three cases is the same; the differing effects arise from the varying amounts consumed and the varying functions and dysfunctions within the users.

drawn, and underactive." The drug brought about improvement in both types, but obviously could not remove the external circumstances that produced their conflicts, and just as obviously could not impart to the child an insight into his or her difficulties.

To explain the "paradoxical effect" of the drug therapy, Dr. Bradley and his associate, Margaret Bowen, reasoned that "amphetamines may well impart a sense of stimulation, well-being, and confidence . . . to a degree that conflicts, though still present, are no longer irritating and distressing."[5] Bradley and Bowen acknowledged that the child's psychiatric conflicts were still present and did not sweep them under the magic carpet of a cure-all drug program as drug treatment advocates would do today.

There may be an element of paradox in the circumstance that Bradley's studies of amphetamine therapy for children pointed the way that the treatment of hyperactivity has taken for the past forty years. Bradley's pioneer study was conducted in a hospital environment. In a later experiment, he and Bowen reported on twenty-four children who had shown and maintained a favorable response to Benzedrine while in the hospital. The youngsters were supplied with the drug when they were discharged, and their parents were instructed in its use. But favorable responses were not nearly so obvious in many of these patients after they left the institution. A number of the children refused to take the medication regularly. The general impression was that in most private homes and average communities, situations that arise are frequently sufficiently disturbing to offset temporarily the effect of the drug.[6] This would indicate that some of the success achieved in the 1937 study was owed to the Emma Bradley Home environment. It would also seem to suggest that Dr. Bradley had little confidence in drug therapy when the medication was left to the parents to administer and the child had to face the realities of life at home and in the community at large. He did not foresee and presumably would not have approved of the present situation, in which nearly a million children — if not more than a million — are living at home and going to school while under the influence of powerful psychoactive drugs. In most cases, such medication is prescribed on the basis of no more than a fifteen-to-thirty-minute office call and routine physical examination. In most cases, also, the prescribed drug is Ritalin, a product closely related to the amphetamines that J. Gordon Millichap places at the top of the "order of choice of drugs" used in the treatment of hyperactive behavior.[7]

The abuse of such drugs by adolescents and young adults during the 1960s received enormous attention from the media. Virtually every newspaper reader and television viewer knew about the amphetamine product "speed" and its dangers. Very few people were aware that schoolchildren in the primary grades were being dosed with Ritalin, which was one of the widely abused drugs. Writing for the highly sophisticated, politically oriented, and socially conscious *New Republic*, Harlan Vinnedge in 1971 thought it necessary to explain the hyperactivity syndrome and its medication to that periodical's readers.[8] The magazine's editors must have agreed that their readership was unacquainted with the controversial syndrome and its even more controversial treatment.

Symptomatic of the general belated awakening to what was happening in the country's schoolrooms, the Health, Education and Welfare Department's Office of Child Development (HEW-OCD) sponsored a conference on the use of stimulant drugs for behaviorally disturbed children. Invited was a panel of fifteen specialists from the fields of education, psychology, special education, pediatrics, adult and child psychiatry, psychoanalysis, basic and clinical pharmacology, internal medicine, drug abuse, and social work.

The HEW-OCD report incorporates much of the myth surrounding the use of stimulant drugs for hyperactive children. The conference recommended that the diagnosis be made by a specialist who would first assess the medical, psychological, and educational resources. It was stressed that symptoms similar to those of hyperactivity may be due to illnesses or relatively simple causes. Above all, the normal ebullience of childhood should not be confused with hyperkinetic behavioral disorders. They noted evidence that hyperactivity is often caused by hunger, emotional stress, poor teaching, and overcrowded classrooms. The report admitted that the dysfunctions range from mild to severe and have ill-understood causes and outcomes, but it was felt that, nevertheless, this should not obscure the necessity of skilled intervention. Medication was seen as a last resort after special education, behavior modification, and family counseling had failed. Drug therapy was not seen as a cure but as a way of helping the child to become more accessible to educational and counseling efforts over the short term. The specialists recommended that drugs be stopped after the child reached the age of eleven or twelve. It was assumed that the physician would adjust the dosage carefully and watch for toxic effects. The conference report went on to say, in response to public concern, that "in the dosage used for children, the question of toxicity noted in the stimulant abuser is not a critical issue; the young child's experience of drug effect, under medical management, does not seem to induce misuse." Fears of medication handicapping the child emotionally "are not confirmed by specialists; under no circumstances should any attempt be made to coerce parents to accept treatment."[9]

What are the realities of the treatment received by our hyperactive children? How often is the diagnosis actually made by a specialist? How many medical, psychological, educational, and social resources are assessed — or even exist to be assessed? Are hyperkinetic behavioral disorders distinguished from disturbed behavior caused by hunger, emotional stress, poor teaching, and overcrowded classrooms? Is medication really a last resort, turned to only after special education, behavior modification, and family counseling have failed? How safe are these drugs, especially when used over long periods of time? How many parents and medical practitioners have mistakenly assumed that these are safe drugs despite the acknowledged side effects of nausea, irritability, insomia, and lack of appetite?

In November 1971 the *Journal of Learning Disabilities* reported that the Bureau of Narcotic Drugs had issued a new order to tighten control of the estimated four billion units of drugs identified as "methamphetamine" and "amphetamine" produced in the United States each year. Manufacturers, distributors, and dispensers were ordered to adopt tighter controls, one of which banned prescription refills. The action was taken as a result of findings that these drugs (1) have a high potential for abuse, (2) have currently accepted medical use in treatment with severe restrictions, and (3) may lead to severe psychological dependence. Fifteen to 20 per cent of the stimulant drugs produced were believed to have been diverted into illicit markets.[10]

Both the FDA and the drug industry have been sharply criticized for the unconcern they have displayed toward their obligations to the American public. One target is the industry's practice of pricing brand-name prescription drugs much higher than generic products though the primary pharmaceutical contents of the two are identical. Sometimes the brand-name manufacturer asserts that his tablet is superior because of a unique combination of basic drug and its carrier material or the tablet's coating. To such claims consumer groups will retort that, nevertheless, the purchaser should have his choice between paying, for instance, $10 for the brand-name medication or $2.98 for its generic competitor. Spokesmen for the industry say that manufacturers must charge enough to pay the costs of researching new products. Critics of the industry reply that drug company research tends to concentrate on evolving profitable, marketable products that will have (or seem to have) therapeutic effects on large numbers of patients — new or improved drugs that physicians will want to prescribe or can be persuaded to want to prescribe.

The manufacturers of Ritalin have been severely taken to task for what Schrag and Divoky call "blatant promotional activities." The willingness of some experts and educators to participate in this manufacturer's advocacy of drug therapy has been sharply questioned. The U.S. Food and Drug Administration has ordered changes in the wording of representations made in describing this stimulant drug. But the FDA, which should be concerned with the best interests of the public, is alleged to weight the scales to the advantage of the drug industry.

Parents should not assume that the FDA protects their child

from dangerous drugs. As Senator Edward Kennedy phrased it while chairing a Senate committee hearing, "The skids are greased" for the approval of drugs for behaviorally disturbed children. Top-level FDA officials support a policy of rubber-stamp compliance when data on a new drug are submitted for consideration. Investigative hearing testimony portrays the department's employees as being intimidated when they attempt to protest the approving of questionable prescription drugs. The burden of proof is seen as resting upon the employee, who might reject an application for FDA approval of a dangerous drug, not on the manufacturer seeking approval of his product. Such is the situation as pictured by journalists and, indeed, as disclosed in official proceedings.

The Senate committee report on its hearings concluded, "The public is at the mercy of careless or unscrupulous drug companies and of family doctors who lack the information to judge the danger and merits of the drugs they prescribe."[12] Certainly the practicing physician is not in a position to sense the out-of-sight perils posed by new pharmaceutical products that have been officially approved but will nevertheless later be found to be the sources of serious side effects.

All the information the doctor has about some of the new drugs may have been provided by a "detail man." Detail men make their rounds, calling on doctors, distributing free samples of new products, serving in part as public relations representatives and in part as sales engineers. One pharmaceutical millionaire has said, "I know that if you call on more doctors than the next man, then you are going to have more doctors writing prescriptions. You have to. Mathematically, it works."[13]

Only recently has evidence mounted to show that hyperactivity is not a mere behavioral aberration of childhood that can be controlled with "paradoxical" stimulant drug medication until, with gaining maturity, the patient sloughs off his or her childish symptoms. That concept is being swept aside as more, and more scientifically planned, studies reveal that a hyperactive child will in adolescence and maturity face even greater hazards than those posed by powerful and sometimes unpredictably acting drugs.

The lesson to be learned from the history of the hyperactive syndrome is that where this syndrome exists there is a hidden, underlying disorder, possibly a mind-crippling or life-threatening disorder. Therein lies the danger. Our hyperactive children live at grave future risk.

3
Who Becomes Hyperactive?

IT IS GENERALLY BELIEVED THAT among kindergarten and primary-grade children, many more boys than girls are hyperactive. The ratios quoted in the literature on the subject range from 3 to 1 upward through 4 to 1, and higher. Why such a disparity exists is unclear, and the question is rarely discussed.

In fact, the preponderance of young males displaying the hyperactivity-with-learning-disability syndrome is a source of embarrassment to most authorities in the field. It is difficult for them to explain the disproportion in terms of sexual differences in little boys and girls who are still years short of reaching puberty. How can we attribute such gross statistical inequality to sexual differentiations that have not yet begun to appear in these children?

Still, it is known that some sexually linked *genetic* differences exist in young children. Most color blindness is inherited, transmitted through the female line but surfacing in the male. The same is true of hereditary hemophilia, the condition of excessive, sometimes spontaneous, bleeding.

St. Vitus' dance occurs more frequently among girls than boys. This is not to imply that any causative factor has been isolated and identified. In both color blindness and St. Vitus' dance, a gender correlation exists. Further, both disorders are within the central nervous system.

To infer that a similar gender relationship exists throughout the hyperactive syndrome would be to advance a hypothesis without evidence — in fact, in defiance of the evidence at hand. In 1975 Millichap published a table of "presumptive causes of minimal brain dysfunction in 100 hyperactive children," which listed complications during pregnancy and at birth, including bleeding, Rh incompatibility, drugs or hormones, toxemia, pelvic irradiation, rubella, and infection, along with prolonged labor, anoxia, prematurity, jaundice, and Caesarean section.[1] In the same year, Dr. Ben F. Feingold advanced his theory that the causes of hyperactivity were to be found in two groups of foodstuffs, the first containing natural salicylates and the second containing synthetic color or flavor.[2]

At this point we must pause to ask: Is there any reason to believe that more unborn male infants than female infants incur birth injuries? Is there any reason to believe that boys more than girls are damaged by salicylates or synthetic additives in food?

To these questions the answer is the same. No evidence supports the thesis that male children more than female children are damaged by these causes. Presumably, there must be other causes of hyperactivity. Consequently, intellectual honesty would compel us to assume that the incidence of hyperactivity resulting from these known causes is shared approximately equally between boys and girls.

On the basis of 3 to 1, one boy's hyperactivity would arise from the same causes as does the one girl's, while the remaining two boys must owe their condition to other, as yet unknown causes. In the ratio of 4 to 1, three boys would owe their affliction to other and unknown causes.

In this last proportion, a population of 1,000,000 hyperactive children would number 200,000 females and 200,000 males sharing the same causative factors, with 600,000 males having some other, unidentified factor or factors of a sex-related nature. Or even as reported in the words of a prominent educator, "Thirty-one of the 32 children in the Franklin County study were boys. The basic reason for this is given as chromosomally sex-linked."[3] (Given, presumably, by the authors of the study, as the writer adds his own comment, "Some consideration should also be given to our society's traditional recognition of boys as more aggressive and outgoing, possibly fostering more activity on the part of boys than of girls.")

Stewart and Olds advance "sex-linked factors" as a "possible explanation" for the disparity in a ratio which varies "from a low of 2.5 boys to every girl . . . up to a high figure of nine boys to every girl."[4] Of course the reader may well question whether boys have in them some factor that renders them more susceptible to the hyperactivity syndrome. Such a factor, if it really exists, would be by long odds the most important single element in the hyperactivity phenomenon — should it be present, eliminate that one and the syndrome would wither away by more than half.

Dr. Charles Bradley in his 1937 report stated that the group he observed consisted of 21 boys and 9 girls and that this ratio approximated that for all admissions to the Emma Pendleton Bradley Home. The experience at the Southern California Neuropsychiatric Institute also parallels that ratio. In later studies, Bradley reported upon groups consisting of 321 boys and 67 girls, and of 77 boys and 23 girls. The Mendelson, Johnson, and Stewart investigations of hyperactive children as teen-agers studied a group of 75 boys and 8 girls. These medical studies are of course statistically minuscule when compared with public school estimates that run into hundreds of thousands, even millions of cases, nationwide.

These national estimates may be projections — for example, on the assumption that there is at least one hyperactive child in every classroom, a figure might be reached by reckoning the number of classrooms. Or a total can be calculated by applying a small group percentage to the whole school population.

Obviously, such projections must fall far short of accuracy in gauging the real situation. Some critics allege that teachers label as hyperactive many boys who are merely high-spirited or disruptive as a result of their ethnic and economic environment.

The effect then would be to exaggerate both the numbers of hyperactive youngsters and the relative preponderance of males as compared with females. It is probably true that teachers lacking training in neurological medicine do make incorrect diagnoses. However, the error may not always be with respect to the disruptively misbehaving boy. Hyperactive girls, assuming their behavior is not so conspicuously disruptive, may escape identification — a diagnostic error that would again tend to exaggerate the preponderance of males.

All we can do is hypothesize:

(1) The number of hyperactive boys does substantially exceed the number of hyperactive girls.

(2) The excess cannot be charged to prenatal or birth injuries, or to salicylates or food additives.

(3) No major physiological predisposition toward hyperactivity or learning disability is known to exist in the male.

(4) The cause or the causes must lie elsewhere.

"Boys will be boys." And boys who won't be boys are in for considerable disapproval from their parents and their peers. If there is a small boy in your neighborhood who prefers playing with dolls to shooting marbles, who would rather dress up in skirts and high heels than wear Levi's with a cap pistol in his belt, you will be aware of some of the pressures brought to bear upon the small nonconformist. Boys in our culture are encouraged to be hardy, brave, stoical, daring, sturdy, and self-confident. As a result, they tend also to be more active, more openly curious, and a good deal dirtier than most little girls. From wrestling in the dirt, picking up and throwing stones, crawling under fences, and eating more windfall apples they become hosts to more pinworms, the eggs of which are easily passed from hand to hand. Little boys also tend to dive into more urban swimming pools and rural, contaminated ol' swimmin' holes, and so to incur more middle-ear infections. They are likely to take more active dares and have more tumbles from skateboards, to be struck severely by more pitched and batted baseballs and icy snowballs, to range farther whether afield or in a metropolitan park, to climb higher trees and fire escapes, to have accidents involving fish-hooks and barbed wire and rodent and other animal bites. More than girls, boys are exposed to trauma resulting from their exploits and misadventures. A small climber's plunge from a tenement landing or the roof of a shed, and the concussion in-curred in that accident, may soon be forgotten. Nevertheless the injury is there and may give way before some later onslaught, as a frayed rope breaks or a bruised tire blows out.

"I double-dare you!" This challenge, coupled with small boys' curiosity, competitiveness, and their natural (and culturally en-couraged) activity and adventuresomeness, combine to tempt them to experiment with sniffing, tasting, or chewing new or unusual substances that can open the way to various addictions, lead or other intoxications, and similar perils to health.[5] Moreover, the young male behavioral code encourages manly fortitude, self-reliance, and a firm-upper-lip attitude of stoical indifference to pain, in consequence of which parents may never be told about episodes of poisoning, vomiting, headaches, or symptoms following head injury.

In today's urban culture, boys are disadvantaged in various ways. There are no woodboxes to be filled, cows to be milked, gardens to be weeded. While very few people today would con-tend that "a woman's place is in the home," a girl's participation in the traditional household tasks may yield a sense both of par-ticipation in the family life and of some preparation for adult liv-ing. For her brother, the traditional rural chores of yesteryear are poorly replaced by Little and Pony Leagues, Pop Warner football, and tennis, all sports in which a minority of athletically talented youngsters do the playing while the majority watch or wander away. Even in an individual sport like tennis, half the competitors are eliminated in the first round of play, and three quarters are sideline spectators after the second round. Small girls' recreational activities, though increasingly threatened, have not been so "organized" and taken over by adults. There are still neighborhood sidewalk and backyard games of hopscotch and jump rope.

Even in the area of psychological hazards, girls are somewhat less exposed than their brothers. Girls are rarely told to be little women, and were they so bidden, the gulf between being a "good girl" and a "little woman" is nowhere as wide as that which separates "a good little boy" from "being a man." Boys are expected to be both "good" and "manly." They are supposed to be kind, gentle, fair, and obedient, yet simultaneously to be hardy, tough, brave, aggressive, and daring; in short, to be both small Galahads and junior John Waynes. The perils of climbing tall trees and challenging the most dangerous surf or ski slope are no greater than the psychological perils of shrinking from such exploits — even in secretly shrinking the boy is psychologically compromised.

Until very recently, the children of broken marriages almost invariably have remained with the mother. There is no father in the home with whom a small boy can identify. Yet the ability of the three-to-five-year-old child to resolve his Oedipal complex or her Electra complex hinges upon the child's coming to identify with the parent of his or her own sex. Here is a minefield of hazard to the young boy.

4

Why General Physicians Are Not Equipped to Diagnose or Treat the Hyperactivity Syndrome

LAURA T.'S ENEMY WITHIN, A CASE HISTORY

Laura T., seven years and eleven months old, an auburn-haired, freckled child, was brought in by her mother because of complaints about behavioral difficulties at school that had started with and continued from the first grade. Her present teacher thought Laura to be intelligent, but totally unmotivated, and too cranky and jittery to settle down to learning anything. The girl was described as being either unable or unwilling to remain seated in the classroom or to refrain from whispering, and in general making a pest of herself. At home, the story was much the same. There Laura was fidgety by day, and at night she had severe problems of sleeplessness.

In the past she had been put on Ritalin, but with uncertain improvement. After one year she developed a facial tic, and the drug was discontinued. She was next placed on a rigid diet, eliminating all food additives, but this regimen was without success in controlling her hyperactivity syndrome symptoms.

Laura's twenty-four-hour day found her going to bed between eight and nine o'clock, having trouble getting to sleep, and then sleeping restlessly. She was often awakened by nightmares, after which she would toss and turn, go to the bathroom, and then to the kitchen for drinks of water. After an hour or more of wakefulness her sleep was resumed. Waking around eight in the morning, she was unrefreshed and grumpy, and dawdled without appetite over her breakfast.

Her developmental history was in no way remarkable. Normal at birth, she progressed normally through the growth phases and early childhood. No behavioral problems were noticed during her preschool years. Her medical history was equally unremarkable. The family history appeared to be of possible significance. Laura's mother had had kidney troubles, and a second cousin had problems with muscle control. An aunt was mentally retarded, and another cousin had cerebral palsy. Thus there existed some evidence of central nervous system handicaps that could have a genetic origin. But Laura's general physical examination revealed no abnormal findings. She was a well-developed, well-nourished child in the 50th percentile as to her height and weight.

In the neurological examination, a good visual acuity was confirmed, and no abnormalities were found in either eye. The associated neurophysiologic examination yielded a normal finding of the brain's electrical wave activity, normal brain structure as indicated by sonar wave investigative exploration, and an only mild abnormality that might suggest inner-ear disturbance.

However, the associated biochemical data indicated a possible allergy or the possibility of parasite invaders in the patient's bloodstream. A Scotch tape anal test revealed the presence of multiple pinworm ova.

Laura was treated with Povan, a vermifuge. She soon began sleeping normally. Her daytime behavior improved as her pinworm infestation was eradicated.

On a number of counts, one may say that Laura is a classic example of the hyperactivity syndrome. First, the child in distress is frequently unable to express in words the subtleties of his or her discomfort to the parents or to the family physician. Laura herself did not realize her pinworms were the cause of her problems, for rapidly growing youngsters lack sufficient experience of a stabilized healthy condition, which is needed to recognize a condition of chronic disorder. Sometimes even well-educated grownups in Laura's situation have had to be told by a physician that their trouble was caused by intestinal worms.

Second, it is not at all unusual for hyperactivity to be associated with sleeping problems in which the child is either unable to go to sleep at a normal bedtime hour, or sleeps in a restless, fretful way with much getting up because of night terrors, sleepwalking, going to the bathroom, or bed wetting. Not surprisingly, such a youngster awakes unrefreshed and is irritable in the morning. The irritability further worsens the youngster's situation, making it harder for him or her to get along with brothers and sisters at home and with other neighborhood children. To top it all off, the child is next involved in deportment and learning difficulties at school.

Third, Laura's hyperactive behavior is more than a simple irritability in response to a pinworm infestation. It is also a response to a central nervous system disorder. The price of sleeplessness or chronic sleep deficiency is chronic fatigue. After a sleepless night, the human body faces the next day's tasks with depleted metabolic reserves and accumulated waste products. The sleep lost is more than a loss of so many hours of rest, for sleep is also a period of repair and growth.

An interpretation of electroencephalographic studies depicts sleep as occurring in two-hour cycles, or patterns, during which three quarters of each cycle is given over to large, slow, delta-wave brain activity (the S-sleep period); the remainder of the cycle is characterized by central nervous system activity and rapid eye movements (the D-sleep period — the dream phase). It is widely believed that the S-sleep is used to refresh the physical person, while the D-sleep is occupied with psychic regeneration. Thus it is conceivable that, with some children, barely adequate slumber permits sufficient rest for the physical self, but the psychological self is shortchanged. Furthermore, in children, sleeplessness appears to inhibit the secreting of growth hormones. (This growth inhibition would, in the light of English research, have been further aggravated had Laura continued her Ritalin medication.)

In addition, certainly Laura's case history is typical of the hyperactivity syndrome in a fourth respect. Hyperactive children are not only unable to cope with their environment by making adjustive, adaptive changes, but are handicapped by their symptoms so that the normal environmental influences cannot work their positive, remedial ways. They are not overactive by virtue of possessing boundless energies; they are a bundle of fidgets, in Laura's case, plunged by fatigue into a condition of nervous instability.

It is characteristic of the hyperactivity syndrome that parents cannot detect the physiological basis of their child's behavior, no matter how hard they struggle to reproach, threaten, and punish the youngster for his or her uncontrolled, random, blundering, seemingly malicious, or apparently just plain senseless actions. This child is unable to pursue a task — it looks like laziness, disobedience, defiance. The youngster is unable to become involved in any activity at home — seems not to care, shirks responsibility, is scatterbrained. In some instances, the child is stigmatized as marauding through the house or in the neighborhood, accused of spiteful mischief, or is labeled a little wild thing who breaks, spills, or otherwise destroys everything he or she touches.

The parents at first see it all as behavior that must be reprimanded by scolding, cutting off allowances, curtailing privileges, or by spankings. But disciplinary measures that are effective with a normal child fail with one whose behavior stems from unexplained, unrecognized hyperactive symptomatology. The behavior continues, and comes to be seen as evidence of character traits.

At this point, it becomes easy for a pathological parent-child relationship to develop, a relationship that will intensify the behavioral problem in the child and will create deepening guilt feelings in the parents, who look to themselves for cause and effect in their progeny. Or each looks at the other accusingly, searching for "how the kid got that way." At some stage of a confrontation with hyperactivity within their family, parents will resort to medical assistance.

One might suppose that any physician in general, family medical practice would be competent to diagnose and treat so simple and commonplace a problem as a pinworm infestation. And so the doctor is, in the context of symptoms that would suggest the real nature of the young patient's difficulties. But, no, all that is proffered the physician is what is proffered in many other complaints of hyperactive behavior and accompanying learning disability or minimal brain dysfunction.

It is true that the family doctor might possibly surmise the role played by pinworms in the child's behavioral and learning difficulties. In perhaps 99 of 100 cases, pinworms would be a wrong guess. There are surely that many other factors that might lie at the root of a child's hyperactive symptoms — for example, various common allergies, any one of which might be the villain.

In Laura's case, physicians had in fact seen this child and surmised that her problem was one that could be managed with Ritalin, or had its origin in food additives.

Guesswork in the diagnosis of hyperactivity proves nothing. The fact that treatment directed to, for instance, pinworm infestation or food additives may be unproductive does not prove that the patient is free of these problems. There is always the possibility that *some other cause* exists side by side with the pinworms and the additives, or with either alone.

A diagnosis that meets these requirements takes far more time than the general practitioner can set aside for any one of the dozen to twenty or more patients seen on an average day. Differential diagnostic procedures also require office space, extremely sophisticated and expensive equipment, technicians to operate the equipment, and, at the top level, qualified interpreters of the accumulated evidence. If these services could be provided by the general practitioner, they would cost many times the specialist's fee simply because of the overhead per case.

The almost legendary skills and insights of yesteryear's country family doctor were acquired in the course of a long practice in a small community, with "Doc" often attending patients through their lives from birth, and along the way coming to know the medical histories of whole families. The families to which children like Laura belong today may enlist the services of an obstetrician, a pediatrician, an eye-ear-nose-and-throat specialist, an ophthalmologist, a urologist, and one or more surgeons. Because of job changes, promotions, transfers, and the need for larger housing, the family may move from place to place, and so every few years turn to other obstetricians, pediatricians, eye-ear-nose-and-throat specialists, urologists, and surgeons. One cannot fairly expect that today's doctors will have the close and lasting acquaintance with their patients that the traditional family doctor possessed.

Nevertheless, observance of the Hippocratic oath and the dictates of simple medical logic require that the symptoms of a patient's disease or disorder must be pursued with vigor to determine what damage they may do, or threat of damage they may pose to the patient's general physical, neurological, and neurophysiological well-being. A further part of the physician's multidimensional approach requires an attempt to characterize the symptoms in relation to their biochemical, infectious, metabolic, or toxic cause. In medicine, treatment can only follow diagnosis and must be governed by it.

The practice of medicine has changed since World War II, and the change has not been merely that doctors no longer make house calls. The era has been one of sulfa and penicillin and their derivative forms, of chemotherapy in the treatment of cancer and of insulin's sophisticated application to diabetes, of vitamins and kidney dialysis, of heart transplants and open heart surgery, of the conquest of poliomyelitis, and of the contraceptive pill. So many victories on so many fronts have created heady expectations within the medical profession, among journalists, broadcasters, and programmers, and in the general public. The patient who once hoarsely pleaded, "Doc, got something for a sore throat?" has lately demanded a shot of penicillin.

Too often, physicians have provided the shot or have prescribed the new remedies being lauded in newspapers and magazines. Doctors have let the routine diagnostic procedures veer away a bit from the whole patient and toward the data supplied by analyses and culture slides. When the patient is a hyperactive child — "restless, impulsive, distractive, irritable, can't sit still" — today's family doctor's diagnosis is too often limited to confirming the existence of these symptoms and thereupon prescribing: "Take two Ritalin daily and see me in three months."

What of the leaders of the medical profession — the makers and shakers of Establishment practices and policies? How was it decreed that a grab bag of assorted symptoms should be lumped together and labeled "hyperactivity"? Who okayed the illogical proposition that symptoms, singly or severally, could be treated with a stimulant pharmacological agent to elicit a "paradoxical effect"? Through what thinking was it concluded that the "paradoxical effect" of calming overactive youngsters by giving them stimulant drugs would necessarily have the further astonishing effect of overcoming also their reading, writing, or arithmetic disabilities?

Appropriate medical measures to be prescribed for a hyperactive child begin with thorough neuropsychiatric examination. Thereafter, treatment may consist in part of medication directed to the control of underlying causes: Drugs may be prescribed to eliminate intestinal worms or to lower blood lead levels or as anticonvulsant measures. In other cases, psychological or psychiatric assistance will be invoked to treat psychic traumas that may be the cause of or among several causes contributing to a child's hyperactivity syndrome.

PART II

SOURCES OF THE HYPERACTIVITY SYNDROME

5
The Search for Underlying Causes

DEBBY B., A CASE HISTORY

Debby at age five years and six months was a small-featured little girl, slight in stature, tastefully dressed, and with long golden hair. She was referred to the Southern California Neuropsychiatric Institute by an educational problems diagnostic service because of her behavioral and speech difficulties. The child's mother, who brought her in, described Debby as a "mean little kid" who had temper tantrums and screaming fits when she did not have her own way. Recently, she had run away from kindergarten several times.

Mrs. B. said that she was exposed to measles three months before her child's birth; she believed this circumstance caused her daughter's problems. Concern had been felt for the little girl from the day she came home from the hospital. As a baby, she cried "continuously," slept very little, did not nap, tired of sucking during her bottle feeding, and while in the crib engaged in head banging and body rocking. Her temper tantrums were an ongoing, almost daily occurrence.

At four weeks she had an oral infection, thrush, manifested by patches of a white, fungous growth inside the mouth. When one year old, Debby had a cowpox reaction after her smallpox vaccination. Each of her diphtheria shots produced severe reactions that required antihistamine medication. From age one and a half on, she had bronchitis chronically during the winter. By the time she was two, a hearing problem was suspected. At two and a half years, she was seen by a neurologist who, without examining the child, felt that her difficulty was psychological. Then she was seen by a psychiatrist, whose evaluation suggested the possibility of infantile autism or childhood schizophrenia.

The family medical history on both sides was without significant health problems, and few definite clues could be found in Debby's own review of systems. Up to two and a half years, she had episodes of choking and gagging on solid foods, and of vomiting during temper tantrums, but she had presented no such problems after that age. She did have a record of bronchitis but none of pneumonia and no current difficulty with breathing during exertion, no blue pallor of cyanosis that would indicate a cardiac problem, and no lapses from consciousness.

During her general physical examination, all of her teeth showed markedly delayed or impaired calcification. Aside from a soft, systolic heart murmur, there were no other evidences of abnormality.

As to mental status, Debby was at first understandably shy, but readily warmed up to the consulting room situation, smiling appropriately and displaying reasonable cooperation through most of the examination procedures.

The neurological findings were on the whole normal. The single exception was that the optic arteries had apparent crystalline deposits along the perimeters, while on close binocular inspection the retina showed what appeared to be a tortuous venous distribution of enlarged blood vessels that resembled pigmentation. A possibility of mixed dominance also existed as a factor in her school performance, particularly in reading. Debby was left-handed, right-eyed, hopped with her right foot, and kicked a ball with either foot.

The associated biochemical data had as its most prominent feature a blood chemistry evaluation showing that Debby's difficulties appeared far more likely to have their origins in a disorder of calcium metabolism than in an interuterine defect caused by exposure to measles.

I recommended further evaluations following steps to control the child's calcium intake and urinary calcium levels. Debby would also have supportive training in speech and reading to assist her in these areas as brain development that had been delayed by the calcium imbalance could now progress and mature.

When Debby was reexamined six months later and the findings reevaluated, I found the heart murmur much more pronounced than when I first heard it. The assessments drawn from the new neurophysiological data were much changed, too. The evidence now pointed toward a lack of oxygenation in the blood supplying the brain. These indications, reinforced by the previously observed retinal vessel engorgement, made me refer Debby to a cardiologist for evaluation of her heart murmur. The heart specialist found that an expanded aberrant blood vessel between Debby's heart and lungs was preventing a normal flow of oxygenated blood to the brain. The condition was so serious as to warrant surgery.

After the operation, the child's recovery was gratifyingly successful. With the elimination of the defect, her hyperactivity, fatigue, and tantrums were likewise eliminated. Soon a teacher was reporting on this little girl's ability to achieve.

If it were not for a multidimensional approach to diagnosis, Debby could have been treated as a hopeless victim of childhood schizophrenia, and in a few years she would have died because of an unrecognized cardiac condition.

Other hyperactive children, hundreds of thousands of them, for lack of such a multidimensional diagnosis, have been treated as if their problem was a malady for which neither cause nor cure could be found and for which the only treatment known to medical science was a stimulant drug.

While much of the physiological, psychological, and technical data assembled in the course of any neuropsychiatric examination must in the end be set aside as not contributing to the ultimate findings, it is still valuable in that it shows what did *not* cause the patient's hyperactivity. As in Debby's case, what has been set aside will later provide the baselines by which to appraise later changes or developments. The *total* multidimensional diagnostic procedures work. Debby was elevated to a level of health she had not previously known, something that years of "alleviative medication" would never have achieved.

Hyperactivity may have its source in obscure, underlying dysfunctions that make diagnosis difficult. This is especially true when years intervene between the original problem and the later recognition of the syndrome. A trauma incurred during infancy can be at the root of behavioral and learning difficulties that go undiscovered until the child encounters the demands and stresses of the schoolroom. The connection is more easily made when the interval between injury or illness and central nervous system disorder is brief. The important point here is that physicians must not be put off because a dysfunction is subtle. Dysfunctions are always subtle in children whose handicapping disability appears as a puzzling hyperactivity syndrome, the nature and even the very existence of which may be in dispute.

While taking the hyperactive child's medical history, the examining physician must be alert to the possibility that the youngster may be troubled by lingering or recurring complications that exist as the aftermath of earlier childhood diseases. Measles, a disease caused by a filtrable virus, may be the precursor to encephalitis, a viral inflammation of the brain and spinal cord, and has been followed by asphyxia and convulsions. Although a measles vaccine was perfected by 1965, and the vaccination protects against whooping cough as well, nearly half of American children have not been inoculated for this common and dangerous disease. Scarlet fever, a streptococcal infection, can be complicated by acute inflammations affecting the membranes of the brain or spinal cord, ear infection, kidney ailment, rheumatic fever, or pneumonia. From pneumonia such complications as bacterial invasions of the heart, blood stream, and central nervous system may arise. Rheumatic fever may also be the forerunner of serious heart diseases. It may occur again and again throughout a patient's lifetime. Or it may in turn be complicated by St. Vitus' dance.

St. Vitus' dance is a central nervous system disorder characterized by uncontrollable spasms (tics) of the patient's face and limbs. While it is not a syndrome paralleling the hyperactivity syndrome, St. Vitus' dance may in superficial ways be said to resemble the syndrome: It has highly visible surface symptoms that are linked to and caused by a central nervous system disorder that in turn is caused by a trauma the patient has suffered or is suffering. Here, by the way, it should be said that, paradoxically, the existence of hyperactivity as a medical disorder may never be admitted by some authorities — because upon its being diagnosed, the underlying cause of the syndrome's symptoms is at once identified and thereafter discussed as a specific, precisely known entity (a cardiac problem, possibly, or a pinworm infestation).

Yet again, neuropsychiatric diagnosis requires taking into account the possibility that any live virus inoculation, no matter how weakened, cannot be absolutely free from some risk of the vaccination causing a persisting, smouldering aftereffect that could, in some child at some critical stage, flare into neural damage — and so be a cause of hyperactivity.

All medical procedures begin with diagnosis. When an unconscious person is brought from the street into a hospital emergency room, the ensuing medical procedures provide a dramatic lesson in diagnostic priorities. The breath of life is the first consideration. Deprived of oxygen, cell destruction and death itself are scant minutes, perhaps only seconds away. Next in order stands the quality of the pulse, for oxygen can reach the brain only by being transported by the circulating bloodstream. Thereafter, injections of glucose and calcium solutions may be given to meet the unconscious person's metabolic needs. Perhaps other treatments will follow, directed to a possible thyroid, adrenal, pituitary, or toxic condition.

The same priorities are observed in neuropsychiatric diagnosis. Here also a search is under way. The culprit sought is the organic or functional problem responsible for the patient's plight. Experience with hyperactive children warns that in these cases several problems will probably be detected.

Perhaps not chronologically the first area to be examined, but certainly the area of first and uppermost importance, is again the breath of life. This the diagnostician views in the wide scope of the human body's use of oxygen in all its complexities. As we discover later, in the case history of Warren M., carbon monoxide toxicity can be responsible for a young person's behavioral problems and classroom failure. Or, as with Debby B., the culprit may be a circulatory defect that impairs the blood stream's capability of supplying oxygen to the brain.

Styles of eating and the character of food assimilation require a wide-ranging diagnostic study. It is said that we are what we eat. It can also be said that what we eat is governed by who we are — our racial and cultural origins, our incomes, our ages. Virtually all children are targets of the junk food industry's multimedia promotion of breakfast, snack, lunch, and convenience foods and ready-to-eat dessert items. Such products in the child's diet are weighted heavily with sugar, salt, monosodium glutamate, artificial food colorings, chemical preservatives, and flavor enhancers. No youngster benefits from a tummy full of dietary trash. Some are made ill by it. Food additives have been accused of causing hyperactivity in at least some children. The inquiries into food habits raise the further question of whether restrictive diets for hyperactive children, excluding many fruits and vegetables, may result in perilously limited nourishment for these youngsters. Also, does the young patient crave sweets or salty foods? Is the child unusually thirsty? Is there an allergy to certain foods, and if so which ones?

For example, the assimilative process by which our bodies convert carbohydrates into glucose, then transform the glucose into fuel and energy, is a very complicated one. A dysfunction anywhere along the line can cause blood sugar levels to be too high or too low, possible clues to diabetic or hypoglycemic conditions respectively.

The dysfunction need not be within the digestive tract. The quality of food assimilation is affected by illness or indisposition elsewhere in the body, for example by eyestrain, headaches arising from a variety of causes, exhaustion, and by a host of emotional upsets, allergic responses, sexual problems, and the reproductive process. Children's stomachs are particularly sensitive to suggestion, and are more prone to motion sickness than adults' stomachs. Vomiting is a very common symptom of the onset of childhood diseases.

Within the digestive tract are numerous possibilities of physiological malfunctioning. A tumor of the pancreas will spur it into producing too much insulin. Excessive insulin secretion can also be produced by liver dysfunction and endocrine disorders or may follow severe physical overexertion. The symptoms may be so mild that their cause is difficult or even impossible to discover. Physical signs may be headaches, dizziness, or general weakness. Or the symptom may be of emotional instability, which in a child may be expressed by the tantrums or the weeping spells that occur in hyperactivity. Yet during a five-hour glucose tolerance test, the patient's blood sugar level may fall a few hours after ingesting glucose, but still stop short of dropping to the extremely low level that most doctors insist on before diagnosing hypoglycemia.

The source of a child's subtle disorder may be in metabolic defects that are congenital. This explains the examining physician's inquiries into the medical history of both parents.

Children need calcium for the growth of good bones and teeth. Calcium also has a role in regulating the heartbeat. When calcium is lacking, the blood cannot begin the process of clotting. On the other hand, blood clotting is possible when no injury requires it, and this can produce a coronary thrombosis or a stroke.

Coronary thrombosis usually occurs in elderly patients. A cerebral embolism is possible at any age, including childhood. The embolus can be any foreign matter circulating in the bloodstream; for example, a blood clot, a fat globule, or bacterial matter. Treatment is preferably by surgery; otherwise drugs are used to dilate the blood vessels and anticoagulants are prescribed.*

Calcium requires the presence of Vitamin D in the body for it to be properly utilized. Also, in the process of blood clotting, calcium ions are associated with Vitamin K in the chain of complex reactions that enter into forming the clot.

Lacking calcium and Vitamin D in the right proportions, children suffer the effects of rickets. But too much Vitamin D can cause loss of appetite, kidney damage, and deposits of insoluble calcium salts in the body tissues. A lack of thromboplastin, a product in the calcium ions and Vitamin K chain of reactions, causes one form of hemophilia, the disorder in which bleeding is uncontrolled because the blood is unable to coagulate.

Serious head and neck injuries occurring in early childhood can underlie later hyperactivity, although these factors are difficult to assess when their influence is contributory and long delayed in being recognized. Recently, I pointed out in the *Neuropsychiatric Bulletin* that subdural bleeding can occur spontaneously (without injury) as well as following either minor or severe head trauma. It can also reaccumulate after treatment by neurological evacuation. The acute picture is one of a waxing and waning of signs and symptoms, particularly with regard to alertness.

To some degree, the whole discussion of hyperactivity's underlying causes applies to the incidence of hyperactivity among American children. Are their numbers increasing out of proportion to their age group's size? And out of proportion to their numbers twenty or thirty and more years ago? The answer, I believe, is pretty surely yes. There probably were more hyperactive schoolchildren in 1970 than in 1950 or 1920. One reason for thinking so is that in 1963, the year in which the 1969–70 first-graders were born, motor vehicle accidents took 43,000 U.S.

---

*It should be noted in this connection that the manufacturers of Ritalin warn that the medication may inhibit the metabolism of coumarin anticoagulants — another indication of the far-reaching effects of this drug, so frequently prescribed for hyperactive children.

lives and injured another 1,600,000 persons, of whom 130,000 suffered permanent impairments and 1,500,000 were temporarily totally disabled. These figures do not include the adults and children who were flung about in abrupt-braking highway incidents in which heads encountered window glass, windshields, and dashboards. Twenty years earlier, in 1943, automobile accident fatalities totaled 24,170. In 1913, the figure was 4,200. More and faster cars on more crowded and faster highways are being involved in more, and more serious, crashes. Thus, in thirty years, the death rate from this cause has risen from 3.9 to 17.8 per 100,000 population.

Cervical torsion injury, commonly called "whiplash," a comparative rarity in the days of the Model T dirt road motoring, now frequently occurs in collisions. Its consequences can be inner-ear labyrinthine instability with dysphoria, with feelings of anxiety, depression, and restlessness, accompanied by abdominal distress with an eye movement disorder (pathologic nystagmus*), which prevents the patient's eyes from tracking correctly and occasions difficulties with reading and writing of the kind of reversals in which "was" is seen as "saw."

This is not to say that dyslexia or agraphia result principally from car accidents. The automobile accident figure is simply one among other statistics. In that same year, 1963, there were 29,000 deaths and 4,400,000 nonfatal accidents in American homes, the victims in many cases being children. Serious injuries originate in home fires, shocks emanating from electrical appliances, kites that fall afoul of overhead high-voltage lines, and the hazards offered by medicine cabinet drugs, garden insecticides, turned-on but unlighted gas stoves, poorly ventilated heaters, power lawn mowers, and chain saws, not to mention bicycle and, more recently, skateboard accidents.

The physical and emotional hazards for children become greater when both parents work away from home — as sometimes they must — and no responsible adult is around to look after the youngsters. Consider the plight of the single parent, as

*See pages 161–162.

a divorced clerk-typist described it in a letter to Anita Miller, who chairs the California Commission on the Status of Women. On a monthly salary of $700, plus $200 from her ex-husband, this mother of three was able to keep her house, buy an automobile, and raise her children until the youngest, at three years old, needed day care. "I can't afford it," she wrote. "I'm facing the loss of everything — even my home — and welfare if I have to quit my job to care for my children. Is anything being done for women who need low-cost, decent care for their children?"[1]

Unfortunately, very little is being done. And the problems of child care do not cease after the preschool years. Primary- and intermediate-grade children also need attention and supervision. Good child sitters are hard to find and keep, and it is harder by far to find an adult or an adolescent who is both willing and competent to look after a hyperactive child. Of course, the best solution — and the cheapest one eventually — lies in treatment that corrects the underlying causes of the hyperactive child's syndrome.

6
Pica and Poisons

GREG K., A CASE HISTORY

Greg, three years and seven months old, with flaxen curly hair and blue eyes, possessed an appealing smile and manner. His third foster mother said that he "would break plenty of hearts when he grew up," and that he would never "stay in one place long enough to settle down to a job and a home."

On his first visit to my office, Greg was accompanied by the foster mother and a church-associated adoption service caseworker. They stated that the child lived in a state of constant motion from the time he got up at 5:00 A.M., with his activity steadily accelerating until he went to bed at 8:00 P.M., after which he remained restlessly awake for another several hours. He did not respond to his foster parents' discipline, and did not get along well with neighborhood children of his age group, part of the trouble being that he chewed on and destroyed their toys as well as his own. For the past year he had been treated with Ritalin, the dosages escalating to 22½ mg daily. Under this medication, his appetite at mealtimes became poor, though he continued to display cravings for unnatural foods.

A neurological examination found Greg to be of average size and agility, with no indication of mental retardation. He was described as an affectionate child, but one who lapsed into very erratic behavior. Although left-handed, the boy showed no evidence of cerebral dominance problems.

The significant clues to Greg K.'s difficulties were disclosed in his random, distracted, and driven behavior, his marked sleeping disorder, and his history of destroying and chewing on his toys, followed by an abnormal electroencephalograph tracing and a laboratory indication of an elevated lead level that was initially 43 mg per cent (normal being 25). Greg was treated with one dose of penicillamine, a chelating agent, with an ensuing reduction of his lead level. Thereafter he was treated with an anticonvulsant medication that helped to stabilize his cortical activity. As a result, Greg's behavior began to improve.

"Pica," is a medical term applied to cravings for unnatural foods. Among children, the habit of eating, chewing, biting into, or sucking on any of a variety of objects, materials, and plants can result in poisoning. Unnatural food craving may be a contributing cause of hyperactivity. The reverse order is possible also. Lead in the environment can pose a special threat to children who are already hyperactive from whatever pathophysiological or psychiatric cause. These children, and emotionally perturbed and nervously irritable children generally, may be the ones likeliest to seek release of their tensions in the practice of pica. An oral satisfaction is involved, as it is in gum chewing and cigarette, cigar, and pipe smoking.

Lead is a particularly dangerous substance that is easily either inhaled or swallowed. It is extremely toxic, and can cause brain damage or death. Lead is a chemical element that the human body is able to eliminate only when it is given medical assistance, and it is one of the known sources of hyperactivity.

Through a study in which hyperactive children were compared with a nonhyperactive control group, investigators found that the hyperactive children had significantly higher blood lead and urine lead levels than the control group. The study concluded that there is an association between hyperactivity and raised lead levels, and this association exists even when those levels fall short of the accepted "toxic range." Further conclusions were that a large body lead burden may exert consequences that have up to now not been realized, that the definition of what is a toxic level needs reevaluation, and that physicians should look for raised lead levels in children with hyperactivity.[1]

In another study, newborn rats that suckled mothers who were eating a diet containing 4 per cent lead carbonate displayed hyperactivity, aggressiveness, and excessive stereotyped behavior at four weeks of age. Furthermore, post-mortem testing showed that lead concentrations in the brains of these young rats were eight times higher than those found in control group subjects.

Such studies provide hope, since by logical inference they tend to indicate that hyperactivity, when it is caused by or is related to lead levels in the body, can be modified and perhaps cured by lowering that lead level.[2] This possibility is, of course, one that the diagnosis, treatment, and outcome of Greg's case history tends to demonstrate.

Lead hazards are abundant. "Premium" gasolines contain lead in a form that can be inhaled around service stations (especially at self-service pumps), tank cars on railroad sidings, near carelessly stored or spilled fuel for power lawn mowers using regular gasoline, and at the scenes of highway accidents. Tetraethyl lead, a colorless, poisonous liquid and an antiknock ingredient in gasoline, can be taken into the human body through the unbroken skin. Ethylene dibromide, another premium and regular gasoline ingredient, combines with the lead oxide resulting from burning leaded gasoline in engines. The combination product, lead bromide, is a volatile gas in automobile exhaust emissions. In Los Angeles, lead is found in much higher concentrations along the freeway routes than elsewhere.

Another source of lead poisoning lies in old buildings or apartments. The use of the crane and iron ball to demolish buildings in the course of urban renewal projects can seed the vicinity with lead particles. Needless to say, the dangers to children of lead-painted residences are immense and are not restricted to any socioeconomic groups.*

Lead-glazed pottery, when used as receptacles for storing or cooking foods, will also be poisonous. Such pottery is no longer commercially manufactured in the United States but may be brought in from abroad or could unwittingly be handcrafted by amateur potters. The U.S. Department of the Interior has mandated the use of steel shot ammunition in certain heavily hunted areas where too many game birds were believed to be poisoned by filling their crops with pellets found around the shooting grounds. The lead "fallout" was estimated at not less than three tons per acre in some marshlands.

Lead pencils, so called, have graphite centers. Still, the habit of chewing on toys and pencils is unsafe because of the risks posed by pigments when these articles are manufactured outside the United States. Children should be discouraged from putting any painted article into their mouths, since they are unlikely to distinguish the highly toxic coloring materials of the adult world from the safer colors of the nursery.†

While the role of lead poisoning in hyperactivity has been increasingly recognized in recent studies and there is mounting evidence that less than toxic levels of this trace element may be causally related to the syndrome, it is not possible for parents, or their children, to live healthily in an emotional atmosphere suffused with fears of and anxieties about all possible hazards. As the medical profession provides services only when called upon to act, it follows that parents — without being phobia-ridden — should be aware of public health agency campaigns and services. In some areas, free diagnostic tests are available as part of a

*Many communities have laws requiring lead-painted buildings to be stripped and repainted if children live there. Your health or housing departments will have full information.

†Among the pigments used in the manufacture of paints are yellow oxide of lead, red oxide of lead, lead chromate (chrome yellow), basic lead carbonate (white lead), ferric ferrocyanide (Prussian blue), and chrome yellow and Prussian blue blended into a green pigment.

campaign against the lead poisoning menace. Ask your doctor or hospital about obtaining them.

Men employed in the manufacture of hats used to sustain central nervous system damage from contact with the mercury used in their trade. The American public was awakened to the lethally toxic possibilities of mercury when, in late December 1969, three members of the same family were stricken with paralysis and blindness after they had eaten pork from a hog that had been fed surplus wheat seed that had been treated with mercury-based fungicide. In the same family, a baby born shortly thereafter was similarly afflicted some months following birth. In Japan and Canada pregnant women ate mercury-contaminated fish, with crippling, blinding, or fatal results to the unborn child rather than to the mother.

Fears grew that mercury wastes dumped into streams, canals, or lakes would, after sinking to the bottom of these waterways, be converted by microorganisms into soluble forms that, after getting into aquatic food chains, would eventually contaminate fish. Mercury, like lead, can inflict extensive central nervous system injury, affect hearing and vision, cause birth defects in fetuses when consumed by pregnant women, destroy brain cells, damage nerves, and sometimes cause death. Early in 1970 the FDA ordered one million cans of tuna removed from supermarket shelves. Public alarm mounted again when in March 1971, the FDA advised the American people to stop eating swordfish, as nine out of ten samples tested contained excessive mercury.[3]

DDT is a chlorinated hydrocarbon compound whose bug-killing properties earned Dr. Paul Muller the Nobel Prize in Physiology and Medicine in 1948. The world's gratitude has turned to dismay as DDT and more recent chlorinated hydrocarbon group insecticides have been found to be toxic to humans and to resist stubbornly being degraded into nontoxic substances.

On June 27, 1976, a panel of seventy-six scientists from eleven countries identified a new source of drug abuse in a group of toxic volatile solvents — model airplane glue, benzene, gasoline, naphtha, methyl ("blue") alcohol, and paint thinner, sniffed mostly by children aged five to sixteen, but increasingly sniffed by adults. Dr. Guido Belsasso of Mexico, a top authority on the subject of solvent sniffing, explained that the practice "can kill and maim. It can damage the brain permanently, soften the bone marrow, and produce anemia, and damage the kidneys and liver." Dr. Sidney Cohen, of the University of California at Los Angeles, said that while "alcohol is commonly cited as the universal and most readily available intoxicant, in fact it is not. The group of industrial solvents and aerosols are even more widely distributed, especially when gasoline is included."

A preliminary study shows that about 1 per cent of juveniles in urban centers in the United States use inhalants. Most of these individuals belong to poor minorities. All of the child "sniffers" surveyed in the few studies made up to now in Mexico, the United States, and elsewhere, suffered from loss of appetite, undernourishment, and damage to internal organs.*

*In 1967 I catalogued the properties, clues to toxicity, unusual clinical effects, the metabolism, laboratory corroboration of toxicity, and treatment relating to toxic fumes and gasses:

Benzene [is] a commonly occurring by-product of naphtha found in the production of paints, dyes, rubber, and in dry cleaning plants. Poisoning usually results from chronic inhalation. Symptoms are 1. headache, 2. irritability, 3. gastrointestinal upsets, 4. loss of appetite (anorexia) and nausea, 5. anginal pain, and 6. vertigo. Signs of benzene poisoning include tremors and fluid accumulated in body tissues (peripheral edema).

Carbon Tetrachloride [is] a common organic solvent used frequently domestically and in industry. Symptoms are 1. confusion, 2. anorexia, 3. nausea, 4. diarrhea, and 5. abdominal pain. Signs of poisoning include optic neuritis, hypertension, and signs of hypoxia. Unusual clinical effects: 1. releases catecholamines from adrenal medulla; 2. decreases hepatic blood flow.

Gasoline, of which it was stated that "recently, inhalation has become a pastime among some adolescent groups." Symptoms include: 1. history of exposure to fumes in concentration greater than 2 parts/1000, 2. headaches, 3. blurred vision, 4. vertigo, 5. buzzing, ringing, etc. in the ears (tinnitus) caused by auditory nerve defect, 6. weakness, 7. restlessness, 8. fatigue, 9. confusion. Signs: 1. ataxia (loss of muscular coordination), 2. abdominal pain, 3. tremor, 4. cranial nerve paralysis, 5. hyperactive reflexes.

Glue (Trieresyl Phosphate) is a solvent of toluene, butyl acetate, benzene. Most active ingredient is organic phosphate, which acts as an anticholinesterase. Used among some adolescent groups for getting "kicks" through inhalation of vapors. Symptoms include: 1. lightheadedness, 2. euphoria and exhilaration, 3. garrulousness, 4. double vision (diplopia), 5. tinnitus. The signs may be slurred speech, lack of coordination, drowsiness or stupor.

Children are susceptible to still other toxicities. The dangers of toluene, the toxic substance involved in glue sniffing, have recently been documented. And there may be a round dozen in that veritable poison chest, the bathroom medicine cabinet.

Like alcohol abuse, the use of marijuana raises debatable issues outside the province of this book. As for hyperactive children, the very questionability of the drug's effects puts *Cannabis savita* among the substances that should be kept out of reach. Aside from the possibility that perception-altering drugs may produce psychosis, it is uncertain how they will interreact with medications. What happens when a youngster who is on Ritalin or Dexedrine or Stelazine indulges in pot? When a child who is under medical treatment for the underlying causes of hyperactivity, and may be taking daily dosages of an antihistamine or an anticonvulsant, supplements the prescribed medication with grass? No one really knows.

These questions are further complicated by the uncertain potency and amount of marijuana used by the child, and the further uncertainty as to possible adulteration of the illegally purchased drug. Finally, the passivity induced by marijuana may make the user compliant to the pusher's suggestion that something stronger be taken.

If indeed there has occurred a dramatic rise in the number of hyperactive children in recent decades, may it not be that increasing environmental hazards are partly responsible? We have seen that lead is a culprit. But why not also mercury, which is capable of devastating central nervous system damage? If mercury, why not also the chlorinated hydrocarbons or the latter-day insecticides attacking the nervous system?

Pica can be the clue to health problems that should be investigated and treated in any case — and certainly before the youngster has swallowed some toxic matter. In addition, whether or not pica has been observed, it is part of good parenting to be prepared to cope with the possibility of a child's involvement in accidental poisoning.

A wise first step is to observe the child carefully, partly to learn whether or not he or she has the habit of biting, tasting, chewing, sucking on, or swallowing non-foodstuffs, partly to make baseline observations of the child's normal behavior patterns. A parent's alert eye will often detect that something is amiss before definite symptoms emerge. Remember the adage that "the patient will tell the doctor the diagnosis"; with small children this can happen only when the parent is a source of reliable information.

In episodes of suspected poisoning, try to determine what the child may have swallowed. Ask his or her playmates. Look for signs about the face, inside the mouth, and on the hands. Smell the child's breath. Observe the size of the pupils. Are there signs of dizziness or nausea? Inspect the play area for telltale twigs, leaves, cans or bottles, and lawn mushrooms.

Officials of the Poison Information Center of San Diego, California, in which wild mushrooms grow the year around, have stated that they get from five to ten calls a day about mushroom poisoning, most of the victims being children. The San Diego County Health Department says that of two hundred varieties of the fungi found in the county, fifty are poisonous. Some poisonous mushrooms provoke symptoms that appear within a few minutes to a half-dozen hours. There are other types whose symptoms appear only between twenty-four and forty-eight hours after the fungi have been eaten. Among the possible symptoms are perspiration, visual disturbances, salivation, tearing, colic, slow pulse, delirium, convulsions, nausea, vomiting, diarrhea, and, with some mushrooms, hallucinations.

Naturally, when one immediately and strongly suspects poisoning, the time needed to make an amateur diagnosis is much better spent getting the child to a physician's office or a hospital emergency room.

Pica may be a serious threat when a child is at the toddler stage, able to get into things but not mature enough to heed warnings. So when a tendency to practice pica exists, the premises should be cleared of poisonous plants. Tenants may not find this feasible, but perhaps the small child can be barred access to the known hazards.

Certainly adults and children alike should learn to recognize poison ivy (*Rhus radicans*), poison oak (*Rhus toxicodendron* in the eastern United States, *R. diversoloba* in the western states), and poison sumac (*Rhus vernix*), all of which are poisonous to the touch and perhaps by means of their smoke when burning. In the annals of toxicology, a classical horror tale is that of the picnickers who died because they roasted their weiners on oleander wands. Whole families of plants, such as the buttercups (*Ranunculus acris*), may be more or less, mildly or severely, poisonous — the Ranunculae include columbine, anemone, larkspur, peony, and, among many others, aconite. The last named is a dangerously poisonous plant that can be used medicinally. The leaves of garden rhubarb are poisonous while the stalks are a common foodstuff. Potatoes are a staple, but the sprouts and the tuber are poisonous when in a green-colored stage.

How does anyone distinguish the toxic from the nontoxic plants? In the words of my friend who gathers wild mushrooms, "The same way you tell a Ford from a Chevrolet, or this year's model from last." Unfortunately, a wildflower that any botanist would declare harmless may be rendered decidedly toxic by an agricultural or garden spray. Oxalis, or "sour grass," which used to delight children with its acid taste and which housewives gathered for dinner salads, is nowadays often doused with herbicide.

Rather than rely on attempts to cleanse the environment of all its hazards, parents may find it advisable to treat the child's pica. Such treatment is feasible if the youngster's craving for unnatural foods can be identified as relating to metabolic problems, or traced to mineral deficiencies, or possibly associated with psychological disturbances. Thus the practice of pica by the hyperactive child may be a symptom that can point toward the underlying causes of the syndrome.

7
Hyperactivity Caused by
Brain Traumas

REGRETTABLY LITTLE IS KNOWN about how many cases of hyperactivity have their origins in blows, falls, tumors, and other sources of physiological, structural damage to the central nervous system. This may be because prominent figures in the field have become accustomed to thinking of their specialty in terms of a disorder that is identified and classified by reference to its symptoms. We find a bellwether authority recommending a particular pill as if the hyperactive condition were always simple and the same, and therefore one medication could be prescribed in every case. Few educators and scientists think of hyperactivity as a challenge to be studied and eliminated by locating and treating its numerous, diverse causes. Rather, the emphasis is on determining whether the hyperactive youngster is "hyper" enough to be pacified with drugs.

It was not always that way. Brain damage gained recognition long before the existence of hyperactivity was acknowledged. The first study of hyperactivity to have a significant impact had as its subjects children who were already institutionalized for disorders ranging from, in Dr. Charles Bradley's words, that of "the retiring schizoid child" to that of the "aggressive, egocentric epileptic child."[1] No matter that we no longer believe that epileptics have stereotyped, egocentric, aggressive personalities. The point is that formerly hyperactive behavior was thought to originate usually in brain damage. Dr. Evan W. Thomas has cited statements from nearly a dozen prominent authorities who, during the 1950s and 1960s, attributed this syndrome to brain injury or damage.[2]

All that has changed. The prevailing attitude now is such that very typical hyperactive behavior, when it occurs in association with obvious brain or nerve damage, will probably never be recorded as hyperactivity at all, but will be put down as an aspect of a particular disease or impairment. We may read in Dr. Dennis P. Cantwell's *Hyperactive Child: Diagnosis, Management, Current Research*, of a classification scheme in which the term "hyperactive child syndrome" may be used only when the child's disorder is clearly not secondary to any other psychiatric syndrome.[3] The requirement seems a long step in the direction of decreeing that hyperactivity exists only when no cause, physiological or psychiatric, can be discovered. In practice, the long step would be toward treating hyperactive children with symptom-masking drugs, and a step away from exploring and treating the subtle causes of hyperactive distress.

The course that the investigation of hyperactivity has taken is not surprising, since the matter is in the hands of educators, psychologists, and psychiatrists whose training has not been in the direction of physiological studies. However, parents of children whose hyperactivity may be rooted in or associated with brain injury or in a disease attacking the nervous system have very substantial reasons for taking an interest in the exploration of physiological factors that can affect the outcome of such injury or disease.

The feelings of helplessness and hopelessness, the anguish and the despair, that are experienced by families of a child stricken by an injury or a disorder directly affecting the brain are tragic. Yet tragedy need not be the outcome, for in the case of a young patient, the presence of a brain injury or impairment is not inevitably catastrophic. In the early years of life, the human brain has potentialities of compensatory development. This is why reading problems caused by cerebral dominance problems can be corrected only in early childhood. As a rule, trauma that afflicts the growing brain of a youngster may go either of two ways. The problem may be resolved simply as the child attains more and more maturity. On the other hand, it can also worsen progressively. Possibly the direction taken will be determined by the medical treatment the brain-damaged child receives. Certainly what that treatment is depends upon diagnosis of the problem, and this with special stress upon the investigation of the physiological environment as provided by the patient's bodily systems.

We may again look to seizure activity (epilepsy) by way of example. This disorder of the central nervous system terrifies the majority of people, even though today medications can control half of the cases and in many of the remainder can reduce the frequency or severity of the convulsions. The petit mal seizures in childhood may, with time and growth, go away. Or they may go into the grand mal variety of seizure. In either event, the outcome will not be written in the stars or be determined by blind fate. The medical fact is that seizure activities are often secondary to a range of pathophysiological phenomena. That is, the convulsions may be caused or triggered by out-of-sight elements, and through comprehensive diagnostic efforts these causes can often be detected, reached, and treated.

Hypocalcemia, a lack of calcium, may be such a factor.

Defective arteriovenous formation, in which the blood moves directly from the tiny arterial exits to the veins, thereby bypassing the capillary field (which should absorb blood to supply nourishment to the cells of the brain), may be such a factor.

Carbohydrate malfunction, with low blood sugar, may be a factor.

A tumor may be the factor.

Infection arising from tuberculosis, from fungi, from whatever source, may be the factor.

High blood pressure may be the factor.

High fever may be the factor.

A deficiency state may be the factor.

Oxygenation problems caused by any circumstances may be the factor.

Bleeding in the brain may occur as a result of accidents in the home, industrial plant, and traffic, in athletic contests, or in cases of criminal assault. Or a lesser contusion may result, or there may be only a swelling. It should be noted that the presence of a swelling, by the pressure it exerts upon the brain, may trigger a seizure. On the other hand, it is also possible to have subdural bleeding that produces only a lethargic response in the patient.

Young children may be decidedly limited in their ability to respond in so many words to inquiries about the location, nature, and intensity of the distress they are experiencing. As shown later, in Victor J.'s case, sometimes a principal, long-lasting traumatic consequence of an injury is discoverable only as it is found in the injured child's behavior.

Differential neuropsychiatric procedures are not limited to determining merely whether or not brain damage or other central nervous system impairment exists. They may be of utmost value in planning the appropriate treatment for the patient. (A course of treatment is not fully appropriate just by virtue of treating the ailment, but by treating the ailment in the light of the individual patient's particular defects and resources.)

Often, the parents of an injured child are confronted with the duty of protecting their youngster's legal rights, and this duty involves assessing responsibility and restitution. Certainly the parents should not agree to a mere token settlement so long as a possibility lingers that ill effects may develop in the future. A thoroughly worked up, widely based differential diagnosis can be invaluable should it be necessary to take the issues of responsibility and restitution to court. For parents, solicitude for the young victim of an accident involves emotional upset, mingling hope and apprehension with uncertainty and exhaustion, just when they are confronted by the obligation of determining the cause and extent of their child's injuries and possible resulting dysfunctions.

8

Depression May Have a Physiological Base

FAYE AND GERALDINE, CHILDREN WITH DEPRESSION

Faye R., seven years and two months old, a white girl, was brought for diagnosis by her parents because of her overactivity, ear sensitivity, and abdominal distress. The parents stated that their daughter changed sharply at about five and a half years, just before she entered kindergarten, when she became irritable, with uncontrolled behavior followed by poor attention span, as if living in a sad daydream. She was placed on Ritalin, 5 mg four times a day, with markedly worse behavior when medication was withheld.

Faye typically went to bed at about eight o'clock without protest. She slept heavily but had frequent night terrors without bedwetting or soiling. Faye also had a history of sleepwalking. Awaking at seven-fifteen, the child was irritable. Her breakfast consisted of cereal, pancakes, and milk. She rode the bus to school. She was given lunch money to eat in the school cafeteria, but usually she snacked from a vending canteen. She returned home between two o'clock and two-ten. The afterschool adult babysitter had recently left because of Faye's tantrum quarrels with her. Faye ate a balanced dinner of meat and vegetables at six o'clock and behaved well after taking her evening medication.

The girl's developmental history began with a normal nine-month gestation. She was bottle-fed and had frequent colic. She sat at four and a half months, stood at eight months, and walked at one year. She declared her left-handedness at age two, when she was toilet-trained. She did not practice pica.

Faye had the usual inoculations. Her medical history included a hypersensitivity to sirens and other high-pitched noises, and it was often associated with stomachaches and nausea. This sensitivity became more pronounced after ear infections at age one. She also had motion sickness and experienced abdominal distress before breakfast. She did not have the common childhood diseases or organic disease, sugar in her urine, high blood pressure, or any known allergy. Her parents were in good health. An uncle, grandfather, and great-aunt had heart disease. A grandmother had high blood pressure.

Faye's general physical examination and her neurological examination yielded essentially normal findings. Her associated neurophysiologic data included an EEG that indicated electrical activity on the surface of the brain cortex. The associated biochemical data disclosed a borderline glucose tolerance result and an elevated thyroid function.

The impressions derived from the diagnostic procedures were that cortical lability (upper brain surface electical activity of an erratic quality) existed, and that steps should be taken to rule out the possibility of a contributing problem metabolizing carbohydrates and also to rule out thyroid abnormality. Toxic reaction to Ritalin was seen as affecting Faye's cortical problem. Reactive depression was associated with the child's physical illness.

Geraldine T., at age eight years and ten months, was brought in by her mother for a neurological evaluation because of her school difficulties and "all-around frustration."

Her mother related that for the past five years Geraldine had episodes of weeping and of violence during temper tantrums. Usually these stormy scenes occurred in the morning. Geraldine had an identified cardiac problem. She had been examined by several cardiologists but with no catheterization. Now in the third grade, she did poorly in math and reading but unpredictably from time to time she would perform well.

Typically, she went to bed between nine-thirty and ten o'clock, and experienced difficulty with sleeping. She had thrashing behavior and was a bedwetter. Frequently she talked in her sleep. Getting up at eight o'clock, she was not refreshed. She had a breakfast of toast and juice and was taken to school by car. She carried a sandwich and fruit for her lunch.

Geraldine's medical history included recent motor therapy. Over the past year she had been treated with Ritalin. There had been a recent four pound weight loss. She was not an itcher, nor was she excessively thirsty. She did have frequent fungus infections and pinworms.

Geraldine is an adopted child, and her natural family history is not known. As for her developmental history, she was adopted at six weeks, sat at seven months, stood at nine months, walked at fourteen months, declared her right-handedness at one year, and was toilet-trained at two years. Her first words were spoken at nine months. She practiced pica. She attended a preschool, an experience described as good. But her kindergarten experience was described as poor.

Inoculation history was diphtheria times three, polio times three, smallpox, measles, and mumps. A test for tuberculosis was negative. There had been no high temperatures with feverish convulsions.

The general examination was noncontributory except for rash. The neurological examination was noncontributory.

The neurophysiologic examination yielded data similar to the EEG and ENG findings in Faye's case, but tended to be more severe in their nature.

The impressions likewise were similar, including mild to moderate cortical lability, which might be influenced by the patient's previously identified cardiac abnormality. It appeared necessary to rule out the possibility of toxic ingestion, occurring perhaps through Geraldine's practicing pica, which could be the cause of her skin rash. Again, depression was associated with physical illness. The recommendations were to stabilize the brain's surface electrical activity with diphenylhydantoin, and to exclude foods with additives from Geraldine's diet.

Both Faye and Geraldine were characterized as having severe sleep disturbance. As skin rashes, intestinal worms, and other irritants were controlled, improved sleep and hence lessened daytime fatigue resulted in lowered irritability and better daytime behavior by these girls.

Depression has long been associated with hyperactivity in children. English and Continental psychiatrists and pediatricians have seen hyperactivity as the child's defense against depression, whereas on this side of the Atlantic depression is more frequently viewed as a result, not a cause, of the hyperactivity syndrome. Four million Americans are afflicted by bipolar manic-depression, a disorder in which the patient experiences alternating phases of nearly frenzied enthusiasm and elation and of morbid dejection and despair. Since both these heights and depths of emotion and behavior originate in the same disorder, we should not be surprised when we see hyperactivity paired with depression in children. Dr. Dennis P. Cantwell relates that he has himself observed several children who developed mild to moderate depressive episodes while they were being treated with Ritalin or an amphetamine. Dr. Cantwell therefore urges that depression should be systematically sought in children who are receiving stimulant drugs.[1]

Monitoring children who are receiving psychoactive drugs is of course advisable. It cannot be done under the conditions that so frequently exist, including minimal diagnosis before prescribing the medication and failure to maintain a schedule of periodic checkups.

An adverse reaction to a stimulant drug is only one of the many causes for the appearance of depression-type symptoms in a hyperactive child. Cerebral palsy, severe mental retardation, and epilepsy have their origins in major traumas suffered by the central nervous system, such as a prolonged deprivation of oxygen during the birth process. Hyperactivity results from less damaging central nervous system traumas. The underlying causes are less visible, perhaps scarcely detectable, and may tend toward symptoms of depression along with indications of behavioral hyperactivity. We should not overlook the possibility that in some children the use of stimulant medications may worsen their tendencies toward depression. From Charles Bradley on, experimenters have observed a minority of youngsters whose condition was worsened by these drugs. A common adverse effect of amphetamines and amphetamine-related medications has been sleeplessness, and sleeping problems are known to contribute to depression in children.

The seeming contradiction when a youngster's behavior fluctuates between depression and hyperactivity does not necessarily point to a cause- (depression) and-effect (hyperactivity) relationship. Both aspects of the young patient's behavior may result from an underlying physiological problem. To emphasize the significance of this statement, I quote from an editorial in the April–June 1976 *Neuropsychiatric Bulletin*, which begins with a quotation from Sir Francis Walshe, M.D., D.Sc.; F.R.S.:

> It is imperative, if the psychiatrist is to achieve an optimal degree of success in the diagnosis and treatment of the psychiatric patient, that he inform himself adequately as to the state of his patient's bodily health.
>
> Some primarily somatic disorders may first present themselves with psychological disorders at a time when no complaints are made, and no signs easily discerned, of body illness, and such subjects may progress to an irreversible dementia if the aetiology of their malady is not recognized, and may be saved from this if it is.
>
> Actually there are many common medical diseases that can masquerade as pure psychological illnesses; from tumors, to diabetes, to pinworms. These underlying disorders, along with their rarer sisters, may co-exist with one another (or along with actual psychogenic problems) and may offer no physical signs or identifying symptoms as helpful clues.
>
> All that the patient or his family may be able to see is a developing

emotional type difficulty, i.e., nervousness, hyperactivity, touchiness, moodiness, apathy, social withdrawal, forgetfulness, distractibility, negativism, truculence. — "G.W." [Associate Editor Gail Waldron, M.D.][2]

Neither physicians nor parents should be content to assign a child's symptoms to "depression" and thereafter consign the depression to "hyperactivity." This only relegates the child to his or her misfortune on the grounds that no cure of the syndrome is known to exist.

The proper course is to relate symptoms of childhood depression to its underlying cause (or causes, as in the case histories of Faye and Geraldine) and push forward to overcome the physiological disorders or deficiencies thus exposed. Then both the hyperactivity and the depression may well be eliminated at a single stroke.

PART III

MYTH, MEDICATION, AND OTHER MODES OF TREATMENT

9
The "Myth" Makers

THE SUMMER OF 1970 MARKED A dramatic and controversial turning point in the treatment of hyperactive children. Thirty-three
years had passed since the publication of Dr. Charles Bradley's
earliest experiment with Benzedrine. During the first twenty
years, stimulant drug medication of schoolchildren remained at
a low ebb. Thereafter began a rising tide in the consumption of
amphetamine and amphetamine-related "smart pills" by youngsters with behavioral and learning problems. Nobody seemed to
take much notice of what was happening. But then nobody
seemed to have noticed the growing number of children who
were caught in the grip of the syndrome.

In Omaha, Nebraska, teachers and doctors, and the families
of some hyperactive children, knew that Ritalin was used in the
public schools, and that in fact the school system helped promote
the distribution of the methylphenidate. Teachers urged parents to enlist their children in the drug use program. The
schools were active in helping parents who couldn't pay obtain
free prescriptions, and the medications were sometimes administered during school hours. In March of that year, a local
medical society bulletin stated that the responsibility of the prescription was not the doctor's but the parent's, and that the parent vested this responsibility in the teacher.[1]

Some parents were indignant when asked or urged to put

their child on medication. Others were dubious, still others, acquiescent.

Suddenly there were storm clouds. A young black woman, a university student and a militant, accused the school board of sponsoring the drugging of school children. A candidate for the state legislature took up the issue. In the nation's capital, the Washington *Post* published the following dispatch from Omaha: "Between 5 and 10 per cent of the 62,000 school children in this city in the American midlands are taking 'behavior medication' drugs prescribed by local doctors to improve classroom deportment and increase learning potential."

Omaha school officials protested. It would appear that the newspaperman had jumbled his statistics. Five years later Dr. Robert J. Havighurst, professor of education and human development at the University of Chicago, told a meeting of the American Association for the Advancement of Science that the 10 per cent figure stemmed from an erroneous newspaper report. Havighurst explained that a congressional investigation had disclosed that 10 per cent was the proportion of children estimated by Omaha teachers to be hyperkinetic, and that very few of these were being treated medically.[2] Corrections do not readily catch up with the shock waves of newspaper headlines. Half a year after its appearance in the Washington *Post*, the mistaken percentages reappeared in the *Evergreen Review* and in *Current*.

For the country's hyperactive children, the Omaha incident was unfortunate. Most people then were unfamiliar with the syndrome. Their likely response to the scandal was: "Five per cent? *Ten* per cent? Oh, I don't believe it! There has to be something wrong." Thus the way was paved for discounting the children's affliction as being fraudulent.

While the summer and autumn of 1970 wore on, members of Congress talked of withdrawing federal funds from schools, of commencing investigations to determine whether any federal money whatsoever had been used in "this monstrous project," and a bill was drafted that would "not only have ended Omaha programs, but also much of the research in children's illnesses conducted by HEW, the National Institutes of Health, and jointly, by HEW, and such groups as the Easter Seal Research Foundation."[3] The effect of the Omaha incident was to focus attention upon a disputed medication while ignoring the plight of the children whose health was at stake.

Even Harlan Vinnedge, who reported the incident and its reverberations in the *New Republic*, could assert that candidate Chambers had opened a Pandora's box and that "irreparable harm has been done to children." The irreparable harm presumably was done by depriving them of Ritalin and Dexedrine. Recognizing the reality of the hyperactivity syndrome, Mr. Vinnedge wrote approvingly of diagnostic procedures that were sufficient to verify the presence of hyperactive symptoms in a child but were insufficient or insufficiently pursued to seek out the underlying causes of the youngster's condition.

The real problems of hyperactive children could not be solved on a political or ideological battlefield. Nevertheless, the lines of battle were drawn. On one side were those who felt that hyperactivity really existed but that it could be adequately treated with Ritalin and similar drugs. On the opposite side was the faction whose members looked upon hyperactivity as a nonexistent disorder (or nearly so) and who asserted that the medications were actually prescribed for the purpose of lulling poor and minority-group children into submissive, robotized conformity.

The position of the latter was reinforced by the publication in 1975 of Peter Schrag and Diane Divoky's *The Myth of the Hyperactive Child & Other Means of Child Control*. This book tends to discredit amphetamine-type treatment for small children, but unfortunately, the two authors, who are not physicians, principally seek to portray hyperactivity as a virtually fictitious disorder. One of their arguments is that "the true hyperkinetic is a rare individual; perhaps one in 2000."

The proffered statistic is based upon two British studies. The first was of two thousand children, among whom the English researchers found only one hyperkinetic child. The second study, of all twelve hundred five-year-olds on the Isle of Wight, reported no cases of hyperactivity. Schrag and Divoky do not tell us how many of the children in the cited studies were medically diagnosed, and by whom, and using what diagnostic procedures. Who were the researchers, their qualifications, and their investigative procedures? How much did they rely on questionnaires, interviews, or tests, and which ones? Moreover, in England and in Europe the terms "hyperactivity" and "hyperkinesis" do not necessarily have the same meaning as in the United States. Indeed, British children diagnosed for "depression" may have symptoms that we in the United States would view as "hyperactive."*

A physician does not know how to diagnose a nation's children en masse. One child is diagnosed at a time, and the diagnostic findings cannot be governed by an arbitrary requirement that one youngster in two hundred shall be stricken with pneumonia, or afflicted by a cardiac disorder, or be hyperactive. Recently in the United States there has been a lively realization that the occurrence of swine flu, or of the Guillian-Barre syndrome, cannot be predicted and certainly cannot be adjusted to conform with the incidence reported in another year or in another country.

Let us use common sense to deal with Schrag and Divoky's assertion that one in two thousand children may be legitimately considered hyperactive. Our U.S. school population is 32 million. That proportion would permit 16,000 truly hyperactive children in the nation. The remainder of our supposed or alleged hyperactive youngsters — and Schrag and Divoky quote an estimate of these children as numbering 15 million — are then to be described as children who face the threat of being drugged, manipulated, and dehumanized.[4] And why? "To serve the purpose of legitimatizing and enlarging the power of institutions over individuals."[5]

To buttress their thesis that hyperactivity is merely an "invented" disease, the authors explain that the term "minimal brain dysfunction" was chosen by a "team of national authorities

*See pages 136–137.

headed by Sam D. Clements of the University of Arkansas Medical School . . . supported by the National Institute of Neurological Disease and Blindness and by the Easter Seal Research Foundation . . . The 'minimal' indicated the absence of extreme behavior, and 'dysfunction' was used to get around the necessity of finding an organic problem."

In contrast to Schrag and Divoky's point of view, a neuropsychiatric diagnostician sees hyperactivity as a chronic disturbance of the central nervous system. The disturbance arises out of such physiological disorders as those that depress the quality of oxygenation supplied to the brain and nerve cells.

Oxygen depletion is in my professional experience the principal cause of hyperactive behavior and learning disability. It occurs in many ways, ranging from faulty heart performance to iron deficiency in the blood. A second and major cause of hyperactivity originates in various hormonal deficiencies and excesses, among them the ones that bring about the body's utilization of carbohydrates.

It may seem an anomaly that deficiencies should cause hyperactivity. But such is the way of the human central nervous system. The agitated behavior of the hyperactive child is no more anomalous than the restless tossing of an adult whose insomnia is worsened by need for sleep. A diagnostician will rarely fail to uncover physiological sources that contribute in some degree to the young patient's difficulties. In any event, there existed no need for Clements and his associates to get around the necessity of finding an organic problem. It is everywhere recognized that hyperactivity can be traced to psychiatric problems in children. It should also be widely recognized that to dismiss serious pathophysiological and psychiatric disorders as mere invented myths will not resolve them.

What Ritalin Can and Can't Do

IT IS TRUE THAT SOME PARENTS declare their satisfaction with the current treatment of hyperactive children. "Why, Ritalin is a blessing from heaven. I tell you, our Henry isn't the same boy when he takes his daily pills." Such satisfaction may arise solely from a parent's recognizing Henry's improved behavior in school. Or, again, the same medication that makes this child quieter and more attentive in the classroom may also be used to make him more docile under the home roof.

Are drugs used to pacify the child, in school and at home, day in and day out? If they are, should they be? May a child safely be kept "medicated" throughout most of his or her waking hours? Here, important practical issues confront us.

There are limits to how many days in the week and how many weeks in the year a child should be subject to the effects of the stimulant drugs Ritalin and Dexedrine. Concerning daily dosage, Dr. Maurice W. Laufer has advised that in addition to the hours the child spends in schools, "ideally, the desired effects should last long enough to cover homework time, without a pre-bedtime-rebound."[1]

Here, of course, the desired effect is ideal from the viewpoint of educators, who are naturally concerned that the child shall complete both classroom and homework assignments. From the viewpoint of the medical profession, it is ideal to restrict the use of these drugs to within the confines of minimal health hazards. Dr. Laufer further recommends, "As the medications control but do not cure and work only for the day in which given, it is perfectly possible and often desirable to interrupt the medication in a number of ways, for instance, omitting on weekends and school vacations."

In practice, his recommended medication would be: "With the amphetamines* available in both tablet and long-acting form, it is most often possible to achieve this with a single morning dose, though some will require a 3 or 4 P.M. dose also. This avoids the handicaps and hazards of administering medication during the school day. Unfortunately, methylphenidate† more often displays a shorter span of action, so that frequent administration may be required."

From the viewpoint of the hyperactive child's parents, the "ideal desired effect" of the medication will very likely not be seen as stopping at school and homework activities. The parent is concerned with peace and tranquility in the home, and with the well-being of the hyperactive child's brothers and sisters. Also, the child's education is not solely a public school responsibility. There are life lessons, attitudes, and disciplines to be learned in the home. If stimulant drugs are appropriate in one learning situation, then, parents may ask, why not in the other?

Dr. Laufer concludes with the recommendation that for those individual children who are disruptive at home, in the neighborhood, and at camp, omitting their medication during weekends and vacations would not apply.

To drug or not to drug? To diagnose or not to diagnose? Surely these questions should be examined in the light of the child's best interest. Every aspect of the situation ought to be reviewed and assessed in the decision-making process. For this to occur, a complete understanding of the prescribed drug and its effects is essential.

A child under stimulant drug treatment, though perhaps no

*Dexedrine, for instance.
†Ritalin.

longer his or her former, hyperactive, distractive, impulsive self, may present other problems — the problems of the too-quiet, overly pacified victim of medication given in larger or more frequent doses than he or she can handle. Also, there is the problem presented by the child who is being kept on stimulant drug therapy even though he or she is not responding to such treatment. It has happened, especially in the instance of therapy without adequate medical supervision.[2]

Under a regulation of the Federal Bureau of Narcotics and Dangerous Drugs, Ritalin can be purchased only by nonrefillable prescription. However, because this drug is made available in containers as large as the one-thousand-tablet size, it could possibly encourage doctors to write larger prescriptions, and hence lead to fewer and more widely spaced checkups.

Of course, virtually any drug may provoke adverse reactions in some persons. The more common, though by no means invariable, side effects of amphetamines and methylphenidate have been listed by Dr. Laufer:

1. The amphetamine look, described as characteristic pallor, pinched facial expression, and dark hollows under the eyes.
2. Loss of appetite.
3. Insomnia.
4. Headache and abdominal pain.

To these adverse reactions should be added continuing losses from normally expected rates of gain in weight and height, which have been found to be significant effects of long-continued medication of children. Dr. Daniel Safer, Dr. Richard Allen, and Evelyn Barr, in an investigation of this aspect of stimulant drug use, found that a group of children who had been on medication for hyperactivity throughout a nine-month school year, but who discontinued it during the summer vacation, showed a summer weight gain rate of 120 per cent of their *expected* gain. A second group, who continued on medication through the summer, showed a weight gain rate of only 60 per cent of their *expected* gain. The first group's summer weight gain was not large enough to compensate for their reduced weight gain during the previous nine months. The study found hyperactive children *not on medication* had percentile height changes significantly above those of children who were receiving continuous medication.[3]

When given in the range of smaller doses — 20 mg daily or less — Ritalin suppressed weight gain much less than did Dexedrine, if at all. Whichever drug was chosen, when large doses were administered the repressive effect on rate of weight gain was the same. The manufacturers of Ritalin state: "Daily dosage above 60 mg is not recommended," and include "weight loss during prolonged therapy" in a list of adverse reactions that may occur.

Ritalin, a product of the CIBA Pharmaceutical Company, a division of CIBA-Geigy Corporation, is the most widely prescribed and marketed of the stimulant drugs that, as a group, have been virtually the *only* medical treatment available to nearly all hyperactive children in the United States. Certainly it is true that some school systems provide special instructional help for youngsters with so-called MBD (minimal brain dysfunction), including small classes, one-to-one teacher-pupil instruction, brief work periods, and immediate, tangible rewards for achievement. But these measures aim at educational goals to be attained despite the disability; they are not designed to eradicate the handicap itself by a process of diagnosis and treatment. Similarly, although a very few children are in the care of clinical psychologists and psychiatrists who do strive to overcome the syndrome, in these cases the effort is directed primarily along psychological lines. Since the nature of educational and psychological programs does not preclude the use of medication, Ritalin is often assigned a role as "adjunct therapy," and so forms a part of the treatment.

In medical journals, the CIBA Pharmaceutical Company has recently advertised Ritalin under the headline THE TREATMENT OF MBD as "an effective agent in the alleviation of the hyperkinetic disorder . . . *Hoffman et al.*, 1974." In this instance, the coupling of the hyperkinetic disorder with minimal brain dysfunction is shrewd merchandising. For in conveying the suggestion that the two disorders are one and the same, there is conveyed the further suggestion that Ritalin, sometimes spectacularly successful in calming hyperactive behavior, will succeed equally well in repairing a learning disability — which, in the light of recent research, is unlikely.*

A suggestion that Ritalin may be an aid in improving scholastic performance may also be seen in the advertisements' use of the photograph of a boy studiously immersed in an encyclopedic book and posed against a section of blackboard. The photograph, reduced in size, heads a second page along with the words "RITALIN (methylphenidate), *only when medication is indicated.*" This second full page is an information sheet addressed to the journal's professional readership. It is of interest to us, first, for what it says; second, for what it does not say; and third, for what it says by inference about the disorder it is advertised to "alleviate."

Here a statement-by-statement analysis of the information sheet may be enlightening to parents of hyperactive children:

INDICATIONS†

CIBA STATEMENT. "Minimal Brain Dysfunction in Children — as adjunctive therapy to other remedial measures (psychological, educational, social)."

Comment. Since CIBA must be aware that "other remedial measures" scarcely exist, this opening definition of Ritalin's indicated role as one of merely adjunctive therapy looks like an understatement of that role.

CIBA STATEMENT. "*Special Diagnostic Considerations* — Special etiology of Minimal Brain Dysfunction (MBD) is unknown, and there is no single diagnostic test. Adequate diagnosis requires the use not only of medical but of special psychological, educational, and social resources."

Comment. The statement is partially in error, for while there is

*See page 91.
†"Indications" — uses for which the product is suitable.

no one individual test for a specific cause of the disorder, there are multiple etiological explanations for so-called minimal brain dysfunction. These span the broad differential toxic, metabolic, postinfectious, structural, and neurological lesions that are frequently diagnosable but are not frequently diagnosed, particularly in instances when Ritalin is used prematurely.

CIBA STATEMENT. "Characteristics commonly reported include: chronic history of short attention span, distractibility, emotional lability, impulsivity, and moderate to severe hyperactivity; minor neurological signs and abnormal EEG. Learning may or may not be impaired. The diagnosis of MBD must be based upon a complete history and evaluation of the child and not solely on the presence of one or more of these characteristics."

Comment. The listed historical symptoms to be considered in diagnosing MBD are lacking particularly the two areas of sleeping and eating characteristics. The quality, duration, and reaction to sleep, and the types of eating and of responses to eating, as observed before and after eating, are of double significance. First, because both areas are highly important in diagnosing and treating the hyperactivity syndrome; second, because Ritalin medication in itself can profoundly influence sleeping and eating patterns. If these patterns are overlooked in making the original diagnosis, then in many instances the child's sleeping and eating traits can in subsequent investigations be precursors to or also involved in presenting symptoms of minimal brain dysfunction.

Again, the statement fails to emphasize the need for baseline blood studies prior to using the medication; such findings are necessary before later periodic blood studies are made. It might be more appropriate for the CIBA statement to say that it is important to establish the complete blood picture prior to drug use, since Ritalin will frequently change the blood chemistries.

CIBA STATEMENT. "Drug treatment is not recommended for all children with MBD. Stimulants are not intended for use in the child who exhibits symptoms secondary to environmental factors and/or primary psychiatric disorders, including psychosis. Appropriate educational placement is essential and psycho-social intervention is generally necessary. When remedial measures alone are insufficient, the decision to prescribe stimulant medication will depend upon the physician's assessment of the chronicity and severity of the child's symptoms."

Comment. This statement, of course, gives priority and emphasis to behavior of a nontoxic medical type, yet fails to take into consideration that children may be getting into difficulty with environmental factors or psychiatric disorders at times when they don't feel well because of some medical disease that preceded the decompensation.

CONTRAINDICATIONS*

CIBA STATEMENT. "Marked anxiety, tension, and agitation, since Ritalin may aggravate these symptoms. Also contraindicated in patients known to be hypersensitive to the drug and in patients with glaucoma."

Comment. Anxiety, tension, and agitation certainly are symptoms consistent with MBD, so called, as being part of the complex hyperactivity syndrome, and therefore would militate against the use of Ritalin in most instances of so-called hyperkinetic disorder, hyperactivity, and the like. Glaucoma as a contraindication is suggestive of the mischief that stimulant drugs, depressant drugs, and the presence of various chemical compounds in the atmosphere or in foodstuffs can work in children. Glaucoma is an eye disease that can cause blindness, and yet is often not discovered until too late. Hence, a condition of early, existing but unsuspected glaucoma might be worsened by the administration of Ritalin for hyperactivity.

WARNINGS

CIBA STATEMENT. "Ritalin should not be used in children under six years, since safety and efficacy in this age group have not been established."

*I.e., conditions under which the drug is *not* indicated.

Comment. Despite this warning, it is a fact that children as young as age three are started on the medication. Dosages ranging from 20 to 40 mg are not infrequently given to children under the age of six. That safety and efficacy for this age group have not been established is of particular importance, since hyperactivity usually appears between the third and sixth years (inclusive), an age group having a high frequency occurrence of the syndrome.

CIBA STATEMENT. "Sufficient data on safety and efficacy of long-term use of Ritalin in children with minimal brain dysfunction are not yet available."

Comment. This is a surprising admission, since many children have been on Ritalin for years, and typically a treating physician will say that the child can expect to come off the medication once he or she reaches puberty, often having started the medication at age five or six.

CIBA STATEMENT. "Although a causal relationship has not been established, suppression of growth (i.e., weight gain and/or height) has been reported with long-term use of stimulants in children."

Comment. It is a well-known fact that amphetamines and Ritalin are appetite suppressants; also, studies reported in England demonstrate there is a suppression of growth hormones.

CIBA STATEMENT. "Ritalin should not be used for severe depression of either exogenous or endogenous origin or for the prevention of normal fatigue states."

Comment. It should be noted that detecting an existing depression, of external or internal origin, in children is frequently difficult because agitation accompanying the hyperactivity syndrome secondary to a basic depression is frequently present.

CIBA STATEMENT. "Ritalin may lower the convulsive threshold in patients with or without prior seizures; with or without prior EEG abnormalities; even in the absence of seizures."

Comment. This may have been confirmed recently in Taft, California, where several children allegedly had their predisposition to epileptic seizures of unknown causes precipitated in relation to using Ritalin.

CIBA STATEMENT. "Use cautiously in patients with hypertension. Blood pressure should be monitored at appropriate intervals in all patients taking Ritalin, especially those with hypertension."

Comment. It is again unfortunate in this context that hypertension and elevated blood pressures are at issue among the pediatric age group, since, in the majority of instances, the child's blood pressure is not monitored before, during, or after the use of this medication.

DRUG DEPENDENCE

CIBA STATEMENT. "Ritalin should be given cautiously to emotionally unstable patients, such as those with a history of drug dependence or alcoholism, because such patients may increase dosage on their own initiative."

Comment. Certainly one of the major criticisms leveled at the use of Ritalin is the escalation of the dosage by the parent of a hyperactive child in order to achieve a desired effect. As with any medication, the imprudent escalation of dosage should be considered as a threat, and careful monitoring of dose response activity therefore must be the responsibility of the physician.

CIBA STATEMENT. "Chronically abusive use can lead to marked tolerance and psychic dependence with varying degrees of abnormal behavior."

Comment. The statement does not exclude the possibility of long-term detrimental effects, particularly in children who take the drug year after year; and certainly both tolerance and withdrawal symptoms can occur. The basic pharmacology for such reactions has to do with the imbalance of the sensitive bioamine system.

CIBA STATEMENT. "Frank psychotic episodes can occur, especially with parenteral [intravenous/intramuscular injection] abuse."

Comment. The medication is one of the drugs used illicitly by teen-agers and others who tend to abuse drugs and take them intravenously to experience their hallucinogenic effects.

CIBA STATEMENT. "Careful supervision is required during drug withdrawal, since severe depression as well as the effects of overactivity can be unmasked."

Comment. This warning certainly indicates a serious threat related to the influence of the medication and its discontinuation, and just as certainly warrants careful consideration by any physician prescribing the medication if, indeed, the patient then must face the rigors of withdrawing it as stated in the drug dependence caution.

CIBA STATEMENT. "Long-term follow-up may be required because of the patient's basic personality disturbance."

Comment. The above statement implies the occurrence of postdrug dependence reactions arising from the use of this stimulant drug.

PRECAUTIONS

CIBA STATEMENT. "Patients with an element of agitation may react adversely. Discontinue therapy if necessary. Periodic complete blood counts, differential and platelet counts are advised during prolonged therapy."

Comment. This precaution is frequently unheeded. It should not be disregarded, since depression of the white cell count and other blood complications are inherent in the use of amphetamines and methylphenidate.

CIBA STATEMENT. "Nervousness and insomnia are the most common adverse reactions."

Comment. In my opinion and in others' this statement should have been preceded by the warning that children with sleep disturbance or nervousness should not be given this medication.

CIBA STATEMENT. "Other reactions include: hypersensitivity (including skin rash, urticaria, fever, arthralgia, exfoliative dermatitis, erythema multiforme with histopathological findings of necrotizing vasculitis, and thrombocytopenic purpura); anorexia; nausea; dizziness; palpitations; headache; dyskinesia; drowsiness; blood pressure and pulse changes, both up and down; tachycardia; angina; cardia arrhythmia; abdominal pain;

weight loss during prolonged therapy. Toxic psychosis has been reported. Although a definite causal relationship has not been established, the following have been reported in patients taking this drug: leukopenia and/or anemia; a few instances of scalp hair loss. In children, loss of appetite, abdominal pain, weight loss during prolonged therapy, insomnia, and tachycardia may occur more frequently; however, any of the other adverse reactions listed above may also occur."*

Comment. In addition to their specific content, the above statements of indications, contraindications, warnings, precautions, and adverse reactions are of more general value in depicting the scope and potency of the medication so commonly prescribed for hyperactive children. That is to say, we have in this drug not only one that does not cure, though it does frequently alleviate, the symptoms of the hyperactivity syndrome, but also one that is a powerful agent, capable of altering the functioning of the central nervous, autonomic, sympathetic-parasympathetic functioning systems with possible spillover into other areas of hormone and bioamine activity (as, for instance, in the case of glaucoma, and in other conditions in which the use of this drug is contraindicated).

Among the stimulant drugs prescribed for children with the hyperactivity syndrome or learning disabilities, Ritalin is thought to pose the smallest and least significant threat of harmful side effects. Even so, few persons who have studied the list of its possible reactions can fail to recognize that it has mysterious and disturbing possibilities for some individuals.

Urticaria: a vascular reaction pattern of the skin, marked by transient appearance of smooth, slightly elevated patches; *arthralgia*: a sensitivity of the joints; *exfoliative dermatitis*: a severe skin reaction where there is loss of superficial skin layers; *erythema multiforme*: a condition of the skin with variously formed papules and macules, which last for several days and are attended with burning and itching (The lesions may appear as separate rings, or vesicles.); *necrotizing vasculitis*: a severe breakdown of the tissues forming the blood vessels; *thrombocytopenic purpura*: reduction in the number of platelets involved in clotting, resulting in a large bruise; *anorexia*: the loss of appetite; *dyskinesia*: jerky, unsteady movements; *tachycardia*: rapid heart beat; *angina*: pain, usually of the heart; *toxic psychosis*: abnormal behavior related to a toxic substance.

The amphetamine group as a whole is effective only within narrow limits. These drugs have calmed the behavior of some children, though not of all. Probably one in three hyperactive children does not respond to stimulant drug therapy to a satisfactory degree. Some of those who at first are responsive will later not be influenced by the drugs. In all cases, the normalizing effect of the medication lasts for only a few hours after the pill is swallowed.

In the schoolroom, Ritalin seems to cause the hyperactive child to become more subdued and cooperative, but it does not bring about a corresponding improvement in scholastic performance. Dr. Gabrielle Weiss has described the surprise and disappointment produced by the findings in a major study of the long-term treatment of hyperactive children with Ritalin. Dr. Weiss and her associates followed the progress of three large groups of these youngsters. One group had been on Ritalin for not less than three years. The second group had been on Thorazine, an antianxiety, tranquilizing drug. The third group was not on medication.

There were no statistically significant differences between the three groups when the children were tested with the Bender Gestalt visual-motor test, Wechsler Intelligence Scale for Children, and for emotional adjustment, delinquency, and academic performance as measured by the number of grades failed. Dr. Weiss, in discussing this outcome, said of herself and her co-workers, "All of us had in general been impressed by the efficacy of stimulants for hyperactive children, and we probably all expected the study to demonstrate a better outcome in the children who had received methylphenidate* than in those who had received chlorpromazine (Thorazine) or no drugs." She called the results "disappointing," and stated, "Although the hyperactive child on stimulants generally becomes easier to handle, his ultimate outcome may be only slightly or not at all affected."[4] Some of the reasons why stimulant or tranquilizing drugs fail to make significant and lasting improvements in children's behavior and

*Ritalin.

learning achievement have been aptly expressed by another observer. In any situation, at school or in the home, the words of Dr. Domeena C. Renshaw, professor of psychiatry at Loyola University Stritch School of Medicine, apply. Medication "cannot provide love, learning, discipline, skills, self-esteem, or a stable family."[5]

As medications, the stimulant drugs are not remedies; they do not cure. The "treatment" they provide consists merely of squelching symptoms, and that temporarily. Sadly, it would seem that the pills that quiet the children have had the side effect of quieting parents and teachers as well, and almost everyone else who is — or should be — concerned.

Today there are more, not fewer, children receiving stimulant drug medication for hyperactivity than there were in the summer of 1970 when the nation was first awakened by the dispute in Omaha, Nebraska, to the controversial use of amphetamines and amphetamine-related pills to calm the behavior of schoolchildren.

In the years ahead, how many children will be fated to endure a disorder for which no one has troubled to seek the cause, or the multiple causes, in order to find a remedy? As one deeply concerned mother has put it, "When outsiders administer drugs to children, their criteria can be short-term and selfish; peace and quiet in class or at home, a less-embarrassing child in a restaurant, and the et ceteras we all know so well. Squelching a child's tics completely, to make it possible for *us* to deny he has a problem in children head-on instead of ignoring, evading, or a club, is as ghastly as child-beating — it's only more subtle and more sophisticated."[6]

Eventually, the time must come when the government, schools, and medical science will unite to meet the hyperactivity problem in children head-on instead of ignoring, evading, or masking it. Meanwhile, parents should not permit their child to be given drugs to suppress symptoms that may mask an underlying major disorder before an effort has been made to explore the child's problem by a differential diagnosis.

11

Legal Drugs Can Be Dangerous

IN LATE SUMMER 1976, newspapers reported that CIBA, the drug manufacturer, recalled 29,000 bottles of a prescription allergy medication because one bottle in the lot had been found to contain Ritalin. This stimulant is a dangerous drug.

An allergy medication, the antihistamine Pyribenzamine hydrochloride, was distributed between January 6 and April 4 of that year, the FDA said in a statement released to the press. The 50 mg tablets of Pyribenzamine were described as light blue in color and imprinted on one side with the number 33. The Ritalin pills, prescribed for narcolepsy, an uncommon disease that causes people to fall asleep uncontrollably, and for hyperactivity and minor brain disorder in children, were of the 20 mg size and imprinted with the number 34.

"A patient who is taking several tablets daily of pyribenzamine could have a life-threatening reaction if he took an equivalent number of Ritalin pills instead," an FDA spokesman told the news service.[1]

Other amphetamine and amphetamine-related drugs too that are prescribed for hyperactivity have powerful effects upon a child's central nervous system, and especially upon the autonomic nervous system. Particularly at the outset of treatment, the child may suffer malaise, nausea, and epigastric distress as reactions to the medication. These facts have long been acknowledged. In the earliest recorded experiment, 8 of the 30 children who were given a first, trial dose of Benzedrine sulfate experienced enough gastrointestinal distress to color all their other reactions to the drug.[2] In subsequent early studies involving the use of Benzedrine and Dexedrine with young patients, the investigators observed such effects as insomnia, loss of appetite, dizziness, vomiting, and peripheral blood constriction as evidenced in pallor of the face, cold hands and feet, and fine tremors of the hands.[3]

As already noted, Ritalin has been found to produce an increase in the resting heart rate, which can lead to tachycardia.[4] Other effects attributed to this drug are shared by the whole amphetamine group: insomnia, loss of appetite, and abdominal pain. Tofranil, one of the drugs sometimes given to hyperactive youngsters, can precipitate difficulty in focusing the eyes, mild symptoms of Parkinsonism, and glaucoma, possible side effects of tremors, *paralytic ileus,* and lowering of the blood pressure. The prolonged use of some amphetamines has resulted in psychosis similar to the paranoid schizophrenia that has been associated with homicide. Chronic amphetamine use can lead to overstimulation of the central and peripheral nervous systems, in turn leading to overarousal, a disruption in attention, and psychotic behavior.

Serious (major) behavioral changes in two children and one adolescent have been observed as reactions to Ritalin, as reported in the *Journal of the American Medical Association* by Dr. Alexander R. Lucas and Dr. Morris Weiss. All three youngsters had symptoms characteristic of minimal brain dysfunction, or "hyperkinetic impulse disorder," for which the drug was prescribed.

After a first week during which she exhibited mixed behavior, a six-and-a-half-year-old girl, the youngest of the three, became extremely restless and hyperactive, then detached and "strange," and on the ninth day of treatment she cowered in a corner, hid in a closet, was apathetic and mute, and to her parents appeared "almost a vegetable," at which time the drug was discontinued. In a few days she had returned to her former, pre-treatment condition but had developed irregular, patchy bald areas on her scalp.

A ten-year-old boy, in his first week of drug therapy, became irritably restless and hyperactive, screamed in his sleep, was red-eyed and appeared wild, complaining of headaches, abdominal pains, and aching arms and legs. Later he described his experience of seeing a rainbow, a whirl of colors, with lions, tigers, and elephants marching around the whirlpool of lights. The aftereffects of his medication included feelings of weakness and depression.

A fifteen-year-old girl, who to control her hyperactivity had been taking 20 mg of Ritalin twice daily since she was nine, took an overdose of the medication with a sleeping potion during a weekend camping trip and had auditory, visual, and olfactory hallucinations.[5]

These were extreme instances. They were also dramatic reactions, and to the families of the children presented very frightening demonstrations of highly adverse reactions that can occur, even from modest, short-term doses of these supposedly safe medications. A patient having years of medication experience can also get into trouble by doubling the usual dose in combination with a sedative drug.

The harsh reality is that hyperactivity is not cured by drugs and does not automatically vanish with adolescence. Dr. Mark A. Stewart has sagely made the point that teen-agers on the threshold of adulthood have to learn to direct their own destinies, and if they depend on drugs, they may never learn how to control their own behavior.[6] A harsher reality is that children who were put on stimulant drug medication in the primary grades are going to find it terribly difficult to abandon this crutch just when they come to face the strains and challenges of adolescence.

Psychological drug dependence is in fact one of the critical health problems of the second half of this century. It was at first ghetto residents, trapped in poverty and hopelessness, and Hollywood's film luminaries, trapped in the search for kicks, who became drug addicts. In the 1960s much middle-class youth was caught in the Haight-Ashbury drug culture, while their suburban parents often were involved in the Miltown-to-Librium quest for tranquility. More recently, the addict ranks have been swelled by professional athletes, forced into highly charged competitiveness, who gulp pregame speed pills. Now we learn that children can come to like and depend on medication, too. They will associate classmate acceptance and classroom success with it. What will be the attitude toward drug use of the future teen-ager, now in elementary school, who is being required to take Ritalin to counter his or her childhood stresses?[7]

The likelihood of abuse of these drugs by the youngster, particularly when he or she reaches the later stages in adolescence, has been largely disregarded by the advocates of stimulant medications in the treatment of hyperactivity. A government-sponsored report on the use of stimulant drugs for the treatment of hyperkinesis similarly overlooked the peril, believing that such drugs were not prescribed for children after the age of eleven or twelve.[8] However, studies have revealed that these drugs are prescribed until the individual is nineteen or twenty.[9]

Dr. Gerald Solomons, director of the University of Iowa's Child Development Clinic, noted another significant flaw in the myth of safe stimulant drug medications, this in connection with a survey that observed that many of the hyperactive children on such medication had been kept on it for very long periods (an average of thirty-three months) without seeing a doctor, and that parents were receiving permission from physicians to alter the size of the dose or its frequency as they saw fit. Dr. Solomons concluded that, with few exceptions, "patients with minimal brain dysfunction on drug therapy are not being adequately handled by the private practitioner." He suggested the creation of regional centers where children suspected of having the disorder could be diagnosed and treated by specialists.[10]

We have noted that many "symptoms of hyperactivity" are actually subjective findings formed and colored by the observer's personal, social, and professional attitudes. Just so with the "improvements" believed to be the results of drug treatment. These, too, can be formed and colored by a teacher's or a parent's subjective attitudes, such as eagerness to see some change for the better, a desperate snatching at any shred of hope, or by the observer's general confidence in the virtues of medication.

Again, the improvement can be real, and yet not necessarily due to the qualities of the drug. Maybe the child is simply responding to the attention he or she is getting. This happened when twenty-three children were enlisted in an experiment at a state school for the retarded. The experiment was planned to determine whether the drug acetazolamide would reduce hyperactive behavior. The double-blind, random pattern procedures were planned so that neither the staff nor the children would know whether the drug given to the subjects was an acetazolamide, an amphetamine, or a placebo. The test allowed two weeks for baseline measures and a week each for individuals to receive dosages of the acetazolamide, amphetamine, placebo, or no treatment at all. Throughout, the children's behavior was studied while they watched television, were in learning situations, and while sleeping. The observers had been specially trained for their task.

Of the four treatment conditions, the acetazolamide reduced hyperactivity the most, but bested the placebo by only the barest margin; while, compared to these neck-and-neck finishers, the amphetamine increased hyperactivity.

The placebo so very nearly outperformed the acetazolamide because, as the report explained, "the activity room data did not differentiate treatment conditions, and we were able to attribute the placebo effect to a response of the children to getting pills on a schedule or a response of the staff to the idea of giving 'treatment' for the disturbed behavior as opposed to sitting idly by unable to act." The report added that the short intervals between the three-a-day treatments caused a bias against the amphetamine, as that medication requires adjustment of dosage and selection of patients according to their individual requirements.[11]

The point here is that improvement credited to a stimulant

drug may be due to a placebo effect induced by psychological processes in the youngster, the parents, and the teacher. It is a point that has not been overlooked by the proponents of medication.

Dr. L. Eugene Arnold, writing in *Clinical Pediatrics*, sees the stimulant-medicating of hyperactive children as an "art." He states that the "psychologic aspects of the prescribing, giving, and taking of medicines are especially important when trying to modify the sometimes emotion-laden behavior of hyperkinetic children. The physician should start by cultivating positive expectations in child, parents, and teacher . . . the child needs to know that better is expected of him now that he has medical help." Dr. Arnold recommends the cultivation of the placebo effect in the belief that the self-fulfilling prophecy of an expected cure will work especially well in cases of hyperactivity.

Dr. Arnold's context makes it clear that he has in mind the kind of young patient whose problems "are secondary psychosocial elaborations of the original neurophysiologic deficit," and he expresses his concern that "complex vicious cycles can result," and that "once these are established, the minimal brain dysfunction can be stricken from the picture [with effective medication] and the vicious cycle may continue unabated, running on the momentum from its feedback mechanism." Dr. Arnold concludes, "For some children, this [placebo] effect may be of more benefit than the pharmacologic effect."[12]

For some children, perhaps, this can be true especially as the drug's effect may be anything but beneficial.

Overlooked by Dr. Arnold is the risk that the drug administered to the child can so successfully mask the symptoms of an "original neurophysiologic deficit" that the patient's underlying problem will never be diagnosed or treated at all.

It is regrettable, but among those physicians who would use Dr. Arnold's highly skilled techniques for enlisting the expectations of parents and children in support of stimulant drug medication, surely some of those will not adequately handle the needs of their patients. The blunt fact is that a drug program, no matter how deftly it is presented, will not repair a cardiac disorder or any other pathophysiological impairment. Certainly healing as an art has a role, but art should not usurp the role of logic, or scientific investigation, or diagnosis and its verification. For too long in the treatment of hyperactivity, the stimulant drugs have been a stopgap, the "medication of choice" when it is unknown what specific malady, infirmity, lesion, or complication is in need of treatment.

When the cause of the patient's disorder is known, and an appropriate course of treatment is embarked upon, then the patient's heightened expectations are indeed highly helpful in hastening progress toward recovery.

Under the heading "The American Way of Drugging," *Society* presented in May 1973 what was in effect a symposium in print that included Howard S. Becker's "Consciousness, Power, and Drug Effects." Mr. Becker observed: "Illicit drug users typically teach novices the side effects to look out for . . . Many LSD users became experts at 'talking down' people experiencing trips . . ." By contrast, he continued, "patients for whom physicians prescribe drugs seldom share a user culture . . . They can experience profound effects without knowing the prescribed drug is responsible . . . The physician himself may not know, since the drug may have become available before the effects had been discovered."

Becker continued by alluding to women who experienced edema (swelling), depression, and vascular difficulties when oral contraceptives were introduced without knowing about undesired, unexpected effects. I see a somewhat parallel situation when parents are put in the position of giving drugs to a child, spurred on by skillfully manipulated high expectations while being left in ignorance of the very serious effects that may ensue and, in fact, most often burst without warning in the first few days, even first few hours, of the medication.

Overly elevated expectations can be harmful in another way. Amphetamine-type drugs may have dramatic results in subduing hyperactive behavior — so much so that little Billy's parents and his teacher are immediately gratified and relieved when he is put on medication. The message as received by the child can suggest: "Take your pill and *be liked* as a good boy." The danger occurs when little Billy doesn't want to rock the boat with the news that his vision still bothers him or that at times he has breathing problems. The child may be afraid that such disclosures will make his teacher or his parents upset with him again.

How can the erroneous belief that amphetamines and amphetamine-related drugs are all but totally safe survive? A clue to this enigma can be found in Becker's description of the way that adverse reactions are communicated in the medical profession. In a study, hospital physicians and clinical pharmacologists were simultaneously asked to report all adverse drug reactions. The two groups made checks independent of each other. From two thirds to three fourths of the adverse reactions to prescribed drugs, verified by the pharmacologists, were not reported by the doctors.

Physicians tended to report those adverse effects in which danger and morbidity were high, and in which the connections between the drugs and the reactions were already well known. Becker concluded: "This means the system works poorly to accumulate new information, although it is relatively efficient in reconfirming that which is already known." Add the fact that a physician's patients do not usually constitute a community of drug users who pool their individual experiences, and Becker saw the result as "a substantial risk that adverse information will never be accumulated."

There is a greater risk. A reticence and reluctance to observe and speak out critically can create reliance on meager, even on insufficient, evidence. In this connection, I suspect that the general belief in stimulant drugs as the appropriate treatment for hyperactivity originated in just such a way. It sprang from a too hasty, uncritical acceptance of conclusions that proclaimed these pharmacological products to have greater curative powers and fewer undesirable side effects than is actually the case.

Allergies and Hyperactivity

HYPERACTIVITY AND ALLERGIES are often found closely associated with each other. Some allergists believe that *all* hyperactivity is rooted in allergic conditions or is simply part of an allergy-tension-fatigue (A-T-F) syndrome.[1] Many allergists look upon hyperactivity as merely a symptom of some, but not all, victims of the A-T-F syndrome. To support this view, Dr. Doris J. Rapp has quoted Dr. Ben Feingold, author of the popular *Why Your Child Is Hyperactive*, as asserting that 50 per cent of the children responding to his "K-P" diet are allergic and need allergy management.

Rapp concedes, however, that Feingold "personally does not believe hyperkinesis is part of the allergic-tension-fatigue syndrome." In his book, Feingold contends that his theory is not based on allergy at all. Though he affirms that allergies may sometimes cause hyperactivity, his K-P diet is founded upon a quite different, salicylate-sensitivity concept.[2]

All of this may appear dismayingly technical. In truth, the subject is not so very difficult. And it is something that parents of a hyperactive child need to become acquainted with in order to chart a wise course to follow with their youngster.

Everyone knows that a child who has measles once will never again be the victim of that disease. This lifelong exemption is due to "immunologic reaction," which refers to the body's way of trying to evict any alien intruder. Any intruder that provokes an immunologic response is called an antigen. In this case, the measles virus, or antigen, is met by defender antibodies in the bloodstream and the capillaries, where a strange naval battle is fought. Reinforcements from the bone marrow in the form of lymphocytes arrive. Gamma globulins, epitopes of molecules, polypeptide chains, rush into the battle. Clones, which are identical cells especially designed for attacking specific antigens, descend in chains from their parent lymphocytes.

After the invaders are overcome, some of the clones remain to repel any future aggression from the same antigens. For thousands of years, such natural immunization was mankind's principal, if not only, defense against ravaging diseases. Lacking such natural defense, whole populations of primitive people have perished from their first exposure to measles and smallpox. Everywhere, children who had not had these diseases were threatened by the dreaded illnesses until man-made immunization was achieved.

Vaccination with live or attenuated (weakened) organisms, or inoculation with killed ones, can serve to trigger and stimulate the antibodies, and thus raise barriers against smallpox, diphtheria, typhoid, polio, and other diseases. Where a choice exists between swallowing an attenuated virus or having the killed organism injected, safety suggests the second. The discomfort accompanying a needle thrust is a small price to pay for immunity from the discomforts of serious illnesses and the peril of disfiguring, crippling, and possibly fatal outcomes.

Within a dozen years, human allergies may face elimination because of current research. The new developments involve a peptide structure that by inhibiting the release of histamines at the cellular level will prevent allergic reactions.[3]

Allergy is an expression of immunologic response. The invading substances are termed allergens; the defending antibodies are termed reagins. The allergen invaders are characteristically less threatening than the viruses and microbes that cause major diseases. While the majority of human beings are not even aware of the existance of dandruff, pollen, mold, and various potential allergens possessed by foodstuffs, these elements can plunge other people into fits of coughing, sneezing, paroxysmal asthma, or acute gastric distress.

One bout with a particular antigen results in lifelong immunity. Not so with allergens. Sometimes, to be sure, a medical specialist can determine the identity of the problem-causing allergen, and sometimes desensitization can be obtained by injections that provoke adequate immunologic response. But the defending reagins, in contrast to the vigorous antibodies that repel an invading virus, can do little or nothing to rescue an allergy victim from assaulting allergens. Instead, the reagins can play havoc with the body tissues they are striving to protect. In less serious cases, hives, asthma, and hay fever symptoms result from the excessive activity of the reagins. The most serious instances of this are observed when hypersensitivity exists to drugs, chemicals, and some infectious microorganisms. Extremely grave consequences follow when a person who has previously become sensitized to such a drug as penicillin receives that medication again.

Allergy can fairly be described as an immunologic process that fails to function successfully. In some cases, the inadequacy of the natural defenses against allergens puts such severe strain upon the central nervous system that hyperactivity occurs. The theory that hyperactivity is "merely part" of the A-T-F syndrome at once raises the question: What *is* the A-T-F syndrome? Dr. Rapp has stated that the syndrome may be detected by the patient's "allergic-looking" face. Such a face is described as having eye wrinkles, black circles under the eyes, puffiness below or lateral to the eyes, nose wrinkles, and being pale, dull, and apathetic. The characterization is strikingly like Laufer's description of the "amphetamine look," a side effect of amphetamines and amphetamine-type drugs.*

Dr. Rapp has also stated that the A-T-F syndrome can be diagnosed on the basis of patient and family history of allergy and by the feeding problems and hyperactive behavior in in-

*See page 82.

fancy, including sleeplessness, excessive perspiration, and strong cravings for certain foods such as chocolate, milk, and peanuts. All of this amounts to characterizing the A-T-F syndrome as one in which the child is allergic *and* hyperactive by definition. But we need to look beyond definitions into the realities encountered in the thorough diagnosis of individual children.

Both the "allergic face" and the "amphetamine look" are frequently observed while examining children who are suffering from insomnia. Sleep problems may arise from the discomforts of allergies, as well as being side effects of stimulant drug medication. But that is not all. Insomnia may also be present as a symptom of serious, underlying physiological or psychological disorders. Hence a warning to the parents of a hyperactive child: In choosing a treatment for your youngster, the allergy-focused approach should not bypass the broad differential diagnosis that can discover the clue to an unidentified, unsuspected organic or functional illness.

The same caution should govern the taking of the family history of the allergic child and the child's own history of persistent allergy. It must never be forgotten that the very obvious presence of some one disorder does not rule out the possible existence of other, far from obvious, but highly significant health problems.

In fact, the very symptoms that apparently point to allergy in an obvious way may really be pointing to something else. For instance: Copious nasal drip would appear to be an unmistakable symptom of allergic rhinitis, and the more copious the flow the more acute the allergy. Yet the possibility exists that cerebral-spinal fluid may be escaping through an injury to the membrane wrapping that envelops the brain, the dura mater. It is a possibility that can be tested by Clinistik for glucose (sugar), the presence of which confirms that the cerebral-spinal leakage exists.

Again, certainly headache may be symptomatic of allergic distress, caused perhaps by eating licorice, chocolate, or by the "Chinese restaurant" (monosodium glutamate) reaction. But headache also may have its source in eyestrain; flaws of the eyes, the ears, or the nose; or in problems with tumors, bone tumors, calcium deficits, sinus troubles, either marked blood vessel dilation or constriction, collagen disease, meningitis, and cervical vertebrae problems. In addition, headache may herald potential etiological influences of a toxic, metabolic, or infectious nature, any of which may be produced by carbon monoxide, nitrates, or by bromides purchased over the counter, or of brucellosis incurred by direct contact with the raw meat or the unpasteurized dairy products of diseased animals. It may be the expression of a psychiatric depression.

The differential evaluation of a hyperactive child's persistent headaches may require the youngster's history concerning migraine headaches; a physical examination that includes blood pressure, spinal fluid, abscesses of frontal lobes, subdural clues, and cortical reflexes; and a psychiatric examination, plus neurophysiological findings — for example, epinephrine activity indicated by ENG examination — with a comprehensive biochemical profile.

Among the common — and often overlooked — causes of headache are temporal mandibular (jaw) joint distress, chronic carbon monoxide inhalation, cervical torsion injuries that left residual effects, sleep deprivation, and various psychosomatic conflicts with respect to pain location and its interpretation.

In prudent medical practice, neither nasal drip symptoms nor headaches alone or together can establish, or serve to confirm, a diagnosis of A-T-F syndrome as being the one responsible entity. For while the child may indeed be allergic to certain foodstuffs or inhalants, this child's headaches may be a symptom of some other serious disorder or deficiency.

What is true of headache and nasal drip applies as well to other signs and symptoms that have been listed as characteristic of A-T-F. There are many causes, some of them extremely serious, for stomachache, leg, neck, shoulder, or backache, excessive perspiration, poor sleep, bladder symptoms, swollen abdomen, rapid pulse rate, irritated or swollen lips, numb tingling of hands or feet, fluid retention, and the more general behavioral symptoms described as fatigue, irritability, eye circles, emotional or medical conditions of hyperactivity, inability to concentrate, or hostility and destructive behavior.

One must sympathize with the desire of parents to find the cause and the remedy of their child's ill health, and yet one must realize that the tendency of A-T-F doctrine to encourage "do it yourself" diagnosis is unfortunate. Equally unfortunate are such popular misconceptions as the idea that allergy is all in your head, or if not there, all in the foods you eat or don't eat. All of this is wrong and doubly wrong when the physical well-being and educational welfare of a child are at stake. In plain words, allergies are real. Allergies are also not the cause of all hyperactivity, or of most hyperactivity. But when allergy does cause a child to become hyperactive, at that point it becomes a crippling disease — a health-impairing, personality-damaging, educationally crippling affliction. The situation is just as serious when allergy by its distracting presence cloaks the existence of other health-destroying disorders. The treatment of allergies belongs in knowledgeable, professional hands.

13

Dr. Feingold's K-P Diet

DR. BEN F. FEINGOLD'S VIEWS on hyperactivity and allergy in children differ significantly from those of Dr. Doris J. Rapp, discussed in the preceding chapter. Dr. Feingold began his career as a pediatrician and later specialized in children's allergies. Eventually he left private practice to join the Kaiser Medical Care Program in northern California as chief of its Department of Allergy.

In 1968, at the Annual Congress of the American College of Allergists, he presented a paper called "Recognition of Food Additives as a Cause of Symptoms of Allergy." Shortly thereafter his basic thinking about allergy changed, and the change altered his concept of hyperactivity. Following the lead of Dr. Samter and Dr. Farr, he switched from a concept of "aspirin allergy" to one of "aspirin-sensitivity." The difference between these concepts arises from defining allergy as a natural body defense. Feingold concluded that there could be no natural body defense against the acetylsalicylic acid in aspirin, and hence none to the salicylate radicals in some natural foods, or to other salicylate radicals in synthetic food flavors and food color additives.[1]

The practical consequences to hyperactive children were tremendous. Feingold believes that most hyperactivity and learning disability in children is caused by salicylate sensitivity. Accordingly, he devised a salicylate-free diet, which with later amendments became the Feingold K-P diet. The diet has been widely publicized as a cure, or at least a control, for hyperactivity, or for hyperactivity caused by salicylate sensitivity.

It is Dr. Feingold's published belief that 50 per cent of hyperactive patients have a likelihood of full response to his diet and that 75 per cent can be removed from drug management, even if full response to other symptoms is not achieved.[2] Of course, the statement is open to technical qualifications. Strictly speaking, the percentages may apply only to the doctor's own patients at the time of writing. What "full response" *is* lacks definition.

Nevertheless, the possibility of treating a child's hyperactivity at home simply by following a diet appeals to parents who hope — and in some cases unhappily need — to manage their youngster's problem without expensive professional assistance. The fact is, and we should face it, books and magazine articles are often perused simply for the hints and tips they may give the amateur home diagnostician.

The issue here is a serious one for parent and child. Dr. Feingold does not deny that in rare instances the source of hyperactivity may be a food allergy in which salicylate sensitivity is not involved. Obviously, a youngster whose hyperactive condition is not caused by salicylate sensitivity cannot be helped by this diet. Well, the child can be helped a little, and show some improvement, if the K-P diet is nutritionally greatly superior to what he or she has been eating. Dr. Feingold frankly admits that there are partial to complete failures to respond to his diet.

Yet a child's poor response to the K-P diet doesn't conclusively prove that the youngster is free from salicylate-sensitivity problems. The poor response may only prove that the parents failed to exclude from the diet all of the foods that contain natural or synthetic salicylate ingredients. Dr. Feingold cites instances in which he checked the food diaries kept by his patients' families and found repeated, even daily, infractions of the diet.[3] No one, of course, checks up on a do-it-yourself home treatment.

So parents cannot know what their child's failure to respond to the K-P diet means. This is a formidable stumbling block for them. Even the child's show of "some improvement" is an ambiguous response. True, Dr. Feingold cites with satisfaction many instances of some, or limited, or otherwise qualified improvement. Remember that he is a highly experienced pediatrician and allergist who has examined and diagnosed his patients. This precaution is something that parents treating their own children are unable to take. The parent must recognize that "half-success" is also "half-failure." The element of failure can be pointing to some cause other than salicylate sensitivity, possibly indicating the presence of an undiagnosed serious ongoing process. If so the eventual costs, both human and financial, may be fearfully high.

Dr. Feingold has urged that if "50 per cent, even 25 per cent," of hyperactive children with learning disabilities will respond to the K-P diet, and can be taken off drugs to lead normal lives at home and in school, the diet's "admitted bother and kitchen nuisance becomes both productive and rewarding."[4]

No one should question Dr. Feingold's hope and aspiration. But for myself, based on my own professional experience, the "even 25 per cent" figure seems unrealistically high. Nothing that I have observed in years of clinical experience with hyperactive patients supports the supposition that anywhere near one fourth of hyperactive children are hyperactive by reason of synthetic or crossover-type salicylate sensitivity. In my judgment, Dr. Feingold's test groups were a decidedly unrepresentative sampling.

In *Why Your Child Is Hyperactive*, Dr. Feingold relates his experience with five of his young patients.[5] The first was a six-year-old boy who came with reports from the University of California Medical Center and from the child's pediatrician. His mother was a "calm and very determined" woman who "hated drugs" and who already firmly believed that what her son ate and drank was the principal cause of his problem. Six months later her appraisal was: "There has been a general overall improvement, but I don't like his conduct at school . . ." She considered in some respects that "although the cause is gone, the action still remains."

Dr. Feingold discussed the case with two colleagues. They were both skeptical. So was he, recognizing that the boy's improvement might have been a psychological reaction to the diet program and to the constant attention and vigilance of his parents. "Yet I was encouraged. *The boy had shown improvement.*" In fact, in such situations the psychological reaction is twofold, influencing both the child's behavior and the parent's evaluation of the behavior. The wish for improvement can be father (or mother) to the observation of it.

With respect to his second patient, Dr. Feingold states: "By now I had begun to reach out for other H-LDs [hyperkinesis–learning disability]. I was not satisfied with accidental encounters resulting from TV interviews." Referred by the Kaiser Pediatric Department, this boy of eight, who had been on Ritalin, was taken off the drug, and after a very erratic three-week interval, at the end of the school term, though continuing to have many problems, he had shown improvement at home and in school and was deemed to be "making it."

The third patient was a "Kaiser" baby, now eight years old. At three and a half years he was put on Ritalin for classic hyperkinesis, was later admitted to the allergy clinic in need of an allergen to control a skin disorder, still later was admitted to that clinic a second time, and at age seven was put on Stelazine. On the K-P diet, he improved so that he was taken off the drug medication, though on eating candy or a bakery doughnut he again became temporarily extremely hyperactive.

A seventeen-year-old was brought in by his father who, though he had heard Feingold speak before a group of parents and teachers about the K-P diet, remained skeptical. The son, who had been making "a steady round of doctors" for years, was now in psychotherapy. After two weeks of dietary control, the patient was taken off drug medication. Though Feingold believed that "only time will determine to what degree he has been conditioned over ten years of hyperkinesis," three months later improvement did continue in this youth.

The fifth patient was an adopted girl of twelve who was referred by a Southern California pediatrician. She had been on
Ritalin three years before and was given increasing dosages with
improvement. Then the medication lost its effectiveness. After
she had been on the K-P diet for two weeks, the pediatrician discontinued Ritalin. His final report was: "She has lost her aggressiveness and is at present quiet and well adjusted to her environment. It is still too early to evaluate her school performance.
However, with the ability of the child to concentrate, this will no
doubt show early improvement."

Remarkable results, these. Or are they, when scrutinized?
Viewed as proof of Dr. Feingold's hypothesis that "diet controls
hyperactivity," the five patients make up a group that is both
small and highly selective.

Selective, first, because the hyperactivity syndrome is a constellation of many symptoms that have diverse causes. The longer a
patient makes the rounds of doctors, the greater the likelihood
that common sources of troubles will be explored and found not
to be the right ones. That increases the likelihood that in such a
patient's case the cause will be a rare and unusual one — perhaps
a newcomer on the medical scene.

Selective, second, since in regard to chronic disorders, the
people who are most willing to try a new treatment are the
people who have already tried the old treatments with no success.

Selective, third, in that an unusual proportion of parents knew
about Dr. Feingold's hypothesis and were sympathetic toward it,
and so they were more likely to embark on the new treatment
with their children. The importance here is that improvement is
not a matter of clearing up a rash or reducing a swelling, but depends on behavior, which is judged by subjective standards and,
moreover, is evaluated by the parent rather than the doctor. If
that parent is against drugs, or for health foods, he or she may
be swayed by an unconscious bias. This predisposition to believe
in the remedial power of a pill or a treatment, even though the
results are somewhat less than expected, contributes immensely
to the placebo effect. It is a phenomenon so universal that every

medical study involving human responses must take precautions to measure and discount it.

Selective, fourth, because eminent medical specialists, whose professional reputations are linked with a particular aspect of therapy — be it heart transplants or plastic surgery or whatever — find patients desiring that kind of therapy coming to their doors. The specialists receive referrals from other doctors or former, gratified patients. They are promoted through media exposure. They reach out to the public. The quick-to-believe rush forward; the doubting Thomases shrug and wait to see.

To my mind, it is also significant that Dr. Feingold's highest ratio of success was with his first groups. I would suggest that as word of a spectacularly successful innovative therapy gets spread about, it begins to attract the doubting Thomases; but these skeptical parents tend to be more critical of the results. At this stage, more families dropping out could be expected. Parents who are either skeptics or less than convinced will probably demand complete victory over hyperactive behavior, not merely a "favorable response." Dr. Feingold freely acknowledges that results are often only to be termed improved, leaving something to be desired, or that, everything considered, the response is gratifying.

The K-P diet is hard to follow. Food labels often defy the shopper to find out what really is in the "certified," "flavored," or "hydrolized" contents of the products on the supermarket shelves. There is no simple way to eliminate synthetic additives from a shopping list that includes any preserved, ready-to-eat, or canned foods. Several chapters of Dr. Feingold's book are devoted to the all-but-impossible task not only of purchasing additive-free foods, but also of finding medicines that are not synthetically colored and flavored.

Dr. C. Christian Beels, a psychiatrist, has reported: "The number of working mothers has been climbing steadily, so that now more than half of all mothers work. For mothers of children ages 5 to 18, the figure is 60 per cent and rising."[6] Certainly the parent working away from home cannot plan and prepare the K-P diet meals and be on hand afterward to observe the child, which is absolutely necessary when testing for tolerance to fruits and vegetables that contain natural salicylates. It is also necessary, when keeping the diet diary, to note *everything* the child eats. This last is essential, since the K-P diet serves not only as a treatment but also as the means of diagnosing the child's food sensitivities.

Great reaction followed Dr. Feingold's second presentation, this time before the allergy section of the American Medical Association's annual meeting in June 1973, with coast-to-coast media coverage. Here, seemingly, was the simple, single cause, the one magic treatment that would banish the hyperactivity menace from the homes and schools of America.

Research following the nationwide publicity that heralded the Feingold K-P diet has left the value of this diet open to question. In a study made by the University of Wisconsin in 1976, teachers rated only 6 of 36 boys on the K-P diet to be less hyperactive, 10 to be more so, and 20 to remain unchanged. But 14 fathers and 13 mothers thought their sons "somewhat improved." In an earlier study C. Keith Conners found that 4 or 5 of 15 hyperkinetic children on the Feingold diet were considered improved by both parents and teacher.[7]

Widely discrepant results in such studies will puzzle only those people who regard the hyperactivity syndrome as a one-cause, one-cure disorder. Observers who recognize that the syndrome can be a symptom arising from any of many physiological and psychiatric disorders or deficiencies will not be surprised that any one treatment is inappropriate and inadequate in the majority of cases.

The publication of *Why Your Child Is Hyperactive* opened the door, through the K-P diet, to self-diagnosis and self-treatment. Surely no one having the health of the nation's children at heart would quarrel with Dr. Feingold's *purpose*. But it is possible — and I think necessary — to question the wisdom of giving the Feingold hypothesis precedence over the established disciplines and procedures of modern medicine. No child has been cured by Dr. Feingold's hypothesis, and no one ever can be; the only positive result from the K-P diet is the relief of symptoms achieved by an unknown portion of the population by meticulously avoiding the salicylates.

That, in my opinion, is what Franklin D. Roosevelt would have called iffy.

What is not iffy is that children, behaving and acting in hyperactive ways and labeled as hyperactive, have been found to have subtle, undetected, unsuspected problems of oxygenation, circulatory impairment, carbohydrate and other metabolic disorders, poisoning of various sorts, traumas, pinworm and roundworm problems, defects and deficiencies and psychiatric disturbances, along with the lingering ill effects of childhood diseases — all of which can launch fifth-column attacks upon and through the central nervous system, and all of which, though they may elude less sophisticated examination, can be detected through neuropsychiatric diagnosis.

I cannot for the professional life of me understand why this kind of differential diagnosis should be made to wait while parents and children struggle through trial and error to solve the mysteries of the salicylates. I feel quite certain that Dr. Feingold himself would not advocate such a course. Some of the children I have seen might have died had they chosen that process.

If I were permitted one suggestion to the parents of hyperactive children everywhere, it would be that they *begin* with the best and most thorough diagnostic examination within their reach. First proceed to eliminate every possible cause that available diagnosis can discover. If none can be found, *then* — with nothing to lose — turn to the elimination dietary procedures for whatever help they may have to offer.

14
The "Patterning" Treatment

VICTOR J., A CASE HISTORY

From infancy through the first five years and six months of his life, Victor was a cheerful, vigorous, friendly boy. He was well liked by his kindergarten schoolmates and already showed some qualities of leadership. Of course, he did have character flaws. His temper could flare hotly, but usually only when the situation made it understandable. Also, he gratified unnatural food cravings by practicing pica.

Then, one rainy Saturday afternoon while sailing paper boats in a curbside rivulet, the child was struck by a skidding automobile. For the next twenty-seven hours he remained unconscious in a hospital. He was allowed to go home after a three-day stay, but he remained stuporous for several weeks. Before his discharge, an EEG was taken and was considered abnormal. Three months later, a second EEG was deemed to be normal.

Some of Victor's symptoms persisted, and in time new ones appeared. A third EEG was at least mildly abnormal. A hearing loss was detected. Pseudoisochromatics testing found mild blue-yellow and red-green deficits in vision. Victor now had a right-hand tremor, a well-healed scar over his left thigh, and a bruise remaining over his left leg.

Reevaluation a half year later found that the right-hand tremor had ceased but that Victor had developed a new symptom consisting of repetitive, compulsive speech verbalizations. He would repeat the same phrase over and over without talking gibberish or making nonsense sounds. He was having poor relationships with his schoolmates and was being sent home frequently because of his hyperactive behavior. A nontender, movable mass had appeared on the injured thigh, and the left leg above and below the knee was significantly smaller than the right. A recommendation that a brain scan be made was repeated and effectuated. The scan disclosed a small lesion involving an area of Victor's left frontal brain lobe.

Victor's case history illustrates the possibility of brain damage with symptoms of hyperactivity. If treated by methods that are based on theoretical concepts, the underlying structural trauma will not be disclosed and the condition of the patient can only worsen.

In these pages, concern is focused solely on the problems of hyperactive children. Medications, diets, physical therapy programs, educational theories and practices, and other matters can be discussed only when they are relevant to the central fact of hyperactivity. By the same token, *anything* that purports to help the hyperactive youngster in some way deserves critical consideration.

The Doman-Delacato treatment is put forward as extending to hyperactivity and dyslexia. We need therefore to explore the nature of the therapy — what it is and what it can accomplish.

The treatment was first presented in the description of a study involving 76 children who had been in therapy during 1956 and 1957 for periods ranging from 6 to 20 months. The mean was 11 months. The patients were from twelve months to nine years old. Their median age at entering the experiment was twenty-six months, so that there were as many entering under two years and two months as over that age. There were 16 in the one-to-one-and-a-half-year group, and 41 in the age one-and-a-half-to-three-year group. Of the 76 enrolled, only 19 were over thirty-six months of age. The children's handicaps included spasms, athetosis,* ataxia,† rigidities, tremor, mixed symptoms, and clinical seizures.[1]

The treatments, physical therapy exercises, were performed in the home with the collaboration of the parent or parents, adult relatives, or friends of the family. The parents were trained by Doman-Delacato, and were required to carry out the program exactly as prescribed, four times daily and seven days a week. A parent had to be present to hold the child's head and to supervise the two assistants. One adult managed the child's left arm and leg, the other took charge of the right limbs. The procedure consisted of moving the child in a manner patterned after the crawling and creeping activities of a normal infant.††

A prominent feature of the program required that the non-walking children (56 of the 76) spend all day on the floor and in the prone position. The only permissible exceptions were to feed, love, and treat the child. This requirement alone would seem virtually to exclude single-parent families, families with both parents working away from home, and the poor living in quarters where floor space is scanty, floors are cold in winter, or the building is infested by rodents or insects.

To supplement its "patterning," or retracing, feature, the Doman-Delacato group includes stimulation to foster children's awareness of their own bodies by means of hot and cold applications, brushing, and pinching. Other phases are meant to provide lateral dominance training and proper breathing to increase vital capacity.

The Doman-Delacato treatment was described to the medical world in 1960 as a physical therapy program for severely brain-damaged children. Though the originators limited their claims to those "achieved in terms of mobility," they also alluded in the

---

*Athetosis: tremors affecting fingers and toes.
†Ataxia: impaired control of voluntary muscular movements.
††In Twynyrodyn, Wales, the parents of a brain-damaged child have enlisted a corps of about seventy helpers who take turns in *twice-daily* sessions of a "patterning" program developed at the Institutes for the Achievement of Human Potential, according to Joan Jennings, a senior editor of *Prevention*. ("Don't Stop Now, Karlie Morgan," *Prevention*, September 1976, pp. 127–132.)

same report to benefits to these children "in the areas of language and affect." "Affect" used as a noun is confined to psychology. It means, first, a feeling or emotion as distinguished from cognition, thought, or action; and second, a strong feeling having active consequences.

Are Doman-Delacato methods useful in treating hyperactivity? Should they be employed? Exactly what benefits in the areas of language and affect have been reaped by young, severely brain-damaged children? What does the area of affect include? For our purposes, it is unfortunate that a second report, which promised to deal with the results achieved in other areas by this program[2] and might have answered some of these questions, never did become available.* Similarly, it is regrettable that the three papers presenting the Doman-Delacato concepts and procedures remain unpublished.

In *Brain Injured Children with Special Reference to Doman-Delacato Methods of Treatment*, Dr. Evan W. Thomas provides a comparatively recent overview of the Doman-Delacato method. Presumably it touches upon some of the subject matter in the unavailable, perhaps never completed, report and the papers rejected for publication. The final chapter in Thomas's book was contributed by Dr. Edward B. LeWinn, who with Dr. Robert Doman signed the letter of protest to the American Academy of Pediatrics Executive Board. Mrs. LeWinn edited Thomas's chap-

---

*In 1965, in a letter to the Executive Board of the American Academy of Pediatrics (AAP), a national association of pediatricians, Dr. Robert Doman, medical director, and Dr. Edwin B. LeWinn, director, the Research Institutes, declared:

We have offered to three separate medical journals papers which present the concepts and procedures of the "Doman-Delacato Treatment of Neurologically Handicapped Children." The editorial boards of all three journals saw fit to reject these papers as being without merit. It would seem to us that the widespread publicity generated by the Doman-Delacato program, and requests to the Academy for an evaluation of the program (your statement) would in themselves be sufficient reason for publication of these articles.

Dr. Doman and Dr. LeWinn wrote their letter to protest against an American Academy of Pediatrics Board statement that asserted that "physicians should make their decisions and recommendations for management of the neurologically handicapped child on the basis that there is as yet no firm evidence substantiating the claims made for the Doman-Delacato methods and programs."

ters in manuscript. Dr. Thomas, Dr. LeWinn, and Dr. Doman, along with Carl Delacato, the psychologist, and Glenn Doman, the physical therapist, were all associated with the Institutes for the Achievement of Human Potential in Philadelphia in the 1960s. During that period Dr. Thomas served as medical director of the Children's Evaluation Institute. His firsthand knowledge of the institutes, and particularly of the Doman-Delacato program, is obviously extensive.

Although the names of three physicians head the list of researchers credited in the 1960 report, Dr. Thomas makes it clear that the principal role in the program belonged to Glenn Doman, not an M.D. Repeatedly Thomas alludes to the Doman-Delacato group as "Glenn Doman and his associates."[3] In a chapter on behavioral disorders, Thomas shows a preference for "brain damage" as the cause to be diagnosed in children who exhibit hyperactivity, distractibility, impulsiveness, and emotional lability, with or without other evidence of organic disorder.[4] He traces this term through successive phases: "brain injury," "Strauss's syndrome," "brain damage," and "minimal brain damage," which he finds objectional. (Yet to come was "minimal brain dysfunction.") In this chapter, Thomas's thinking is in line with that of Doman and Delacato. He contends that a hyperactive condition caused by organic damage might be expected to respond to the "patterning" treatment. Thomas defines dyslexia to mean a reading disorder caused by neurological dysfunction that may be genetic or acquired *in utero,* at birth, or later. He states that Delacato brought the same approach to the diagnosis of reading disorders that they used to diagnose children with neuromotor and sensory dysfunctions due to brain injury.[5]

The Doman-Delacato report relied heavily on statistical interpretations in claiming a successful outcome for the 1956–1957 experiments. But how does one measure the improvement in young, severely handicapped children's "motility, language, manual, visual, auditory, and tactile" competence? Since the patients are handicapped, the ordinary standards do not apply. Since they vary in the nature, degree, and severity of their individual departures from the normal, no common yardstick will apply. And, assuming that you have nevertheless measured the amount of improvement in each case, how do you further determine how much of that improvement is the result simply of growth during the period of treatment? How much is incontestably owing to the treatment itself?

Dr. Thomas devotes one chapter in his book to the manner in which Glenn Doman and his colleagues devised the Doman-Delacato Developmental Profile as the yardstick — or slide rule — with which to compute evaluative ratings.[6] Still, there was one big factor it could not calculate. As Dr. Virginia Apgar stated, "Many very young children have symptoms suggesting cerebral palsy during the first year of life, but these symptoms gradually disappear, and by the age of three or four, some of these youngsters appear to be quite normal."[7]

Dr. Apgar bore one of the better-known names in pediatrics. She devised the Apgar Score, an acronymic clinical rating on a 0 to 2 basis of the newborn infant's vital signs. Her book, *Is My Baby All Right?*, is an excellent and comprehensive source regarding such infant afflictions as cerebral palsy, a disorder caused by brain injury usually occurring during the birth process. Obviously, a spontaneous recovery from cerebral palsy or apparent cerebral palsy would vastly damage the reliability of any computation purporting to prove the efficacy of a treatment.

Indeed, Dr. Thomas concluded in the course of his discussion of evaluative ratings that "no statistical method can control the variables in treatment programs which must be carried out in outpatient clinics or in homes over long periods. Nor can statistics provide very valuable estimates of any method of treating brain injured children if the intangibles and uncontrolled variables are given their due."[8] In the light of this statement, we must discount the claims made in the Doman-Delacato report.

The foregoing are the limitations of the Development Profile as perceived by a friendly observer. There may be other shortcomings in the statistics quoted in the 1960 presentation. The report stated that every child seen in the Children's Clinic was included in the study — provided certain criteria were met, one of which was that the child have "a minimum six months' treatment." The report does not disclose how many children may have been entered in the experiment, only to be withdrawn before completing a half-year of treatment because the parents found the program ineffectual and felt it did not justify the efforts required. Speculation naturally arises as to what extent the program — just because of the heavy burden it places on parents, relatives, and friends — tends to confine itself to the more successful cases.

There is another aspect to consider. Dr. Thomas several times seems almost to suggest that parents may derive more benefit from the Doman-Delacato experience than the child being treated. The shattering impact on a family of having a child with a birth defect is known to pediatricians and family physicians everywhere. The frequency with which the blow is accompanied by profound feelings of guilt, shame, and self-reproach is equally familiar to psychiatrists, psychologists, and counselors. The Doman-Delacato methods no doubt do sometimes give parents an outlet through which literally they can work off these emotional states. It is essential, however, that such parental relief is not purchased at the expense of the handicapped child.

The Doman-Delacato treatment remains today what it was at its beginning — a program of arduous physical therapy. Creeping and crawling continue to make up a major part of the treatment prescribed for children with brain injury. Fluid intake is kept at 20 ounces or less in most children under eight years of age unless contraindicated.

Certainly excessive thirst in a hyperactive child may be a significant symptom. But the response should not be to limit the child's fluid intake. Rather, the excessive thirst should be recognized as a possible clue to an underlying disorder; perhaps it points to a carbohydrate difficulty that may also be the cause, or one of the causes, of the hyperactivity syndrome.

The Doman-Delacato therapy is flawed by its fundamental concept of treating *all* patients with *one* regimen. In all cases that involve hyperactivity, parents should be advised to turn away from any therapy that is not related to the child's actual, individual condition, *but that instead is a therapy determined by a theory in the therapist's head*. Children who have a brain injury are by no means immune to other disorders, organic or metabolic or psychological or whatever. Parents who seek to rescue a child from hyperactivity and disability should scrutinize therapies. Will the therapy pay due attention to possible nonstructural causes and contributory factors? What of the psychological and psychiatric problems that may need to be investigated? The biochemical aspects? The toxic? The metabolic? The postinfectious? The degenerative? The submicroscopic?

Parents in whose child structural brain injury and damage do exist should know that modern and sophisticated medicine is not limited to a conjectural diagnosis reared on a foundation of theoretical assumptions. The neurological specialist of today has within his or her reach the capabilities of extremely sophisticated equipment. Medical science has passed beyond its crawling and creeping stage.

15
Coffee

IN RECENT YEARS, TWO CUPS OF COFFEE a day, one at breakfast and the other at lunch, have been tested as a substitute for Ritalin and Dexedrine in the treatment of hyperactive children. One hesitates to use the word "treatment" in this connection, out of respect for its dictionary definition — "the application of remedies with the object of effecting a cure." None of these stimulants can be described as a remedy capable of curing the hyperactive disorder. The realistic and appropriate term would be "symptom-pacifying management of hyperactive children."

As a symptom-pacifying agent, coffee qualifies because it contains caffeine, a stimulant alkaloid that affects the human central nervous system somewhat like the amphetamine-type drugs. There are, however, important differences, both obvious and subtle.

One important difference is that Ritalin and Dexedrine can have more immediately noticed, severe side effects than has the caffeine in coffee, as measured in two investigations. The first study was made by Dr. Robert C. Schnackenberg, chief of the Child and Adolescent Service at William S. Hall Psychiatric Institute, Columbia, South Carolina.[1] Dr. Schnackenberg's account of his experiment made it quite clear that he was not in the least motivated by any prejudice against the two stimulant drugs. He regularly prescribed Ritalin for his hyperactive young patients.

The dissatisfaction with the medication was expressed by the parents of eleven of these children, who were suffering unpleasant side effects. Three had insomnia. Eight had loss of appetite, and among them, two gained no weight and three lost weight. Dr. Schnackenberg's report mentioned other side effects of nervousness and abdominal pain as reasons for parents balking at giving their children amphetamine-type medication.

A pilot study was embarked upon, using coffee instead of the stimulant tablets. The annoying side effects disappeared, and no new ones were noted that could be traced to caffeine in the daily two cups of coffee. In addition to these gratifying outcomes, Dr. Schnackenberg observed no difference between the progress of the eleven children and that of approximately three hundred others he had treated with Ritalin or Dexedrine. As judged by their teachers, using the Davids Rating Scale for Hyperkinesis, the eleven youngsters while on coffee were somewhat improved over what their showing had been while on Ritalin medication.

Technical flaws marred the Schnackenberg study, a principal one being that the amount of caffeine in a cup of coffee may differ widely from any assumed standard. Dr. Schnackenberg himself suggested that a future study should be made, using citrated caffeine tablets in a double-blind, crossover investigation comparing the effectiveness of caffeine with that of some of the principal medications used in the management of hyperactive children.

But there are more serious faults. A false impression of the safety of caffeine is created by measuring it against such dangerous drugs as Ritalin and Dexedrine. The 200 to 300 mg of caffeine contained in two cups of coffee may be augmented by the patient taking an extra cup of the brew, a couple of aspirin tablets for the resulting caffeine headache, and a cola drink — in all, 550 mg of caffeine in less than one day, a dangerous level, equal to drinking five cups of coffee.

The most significant defect is the high probability that the real cause of the child's hyperactivity will remain undiagnosed and untreated and may even be aggravated by coffee consumption.

Unfortunately, the availability of coffee opens the door to the probability of some parents attempting unsupervised medication of their child even in the presence of serious complications; for example, the presence of undiagnosed and unsuspected lead poisoning in the youngster.

A more recent comparison of the relative therapeutic effects of caffeine with those of the stimulant drugs is the study by three Canadian researchers, Dr. Barry D. Garfinkel, Dr. Christopher D. Webster, and Leon Sloman.[2] In a double-blind, crossover study of eight children with minimal brain dysfunction, they found 20 mg of Ritalin daily to be significantly better than 160 mg of caffeine in controlling "impulsivity and hyperactivity."

At the end of the nine-week study, each child had been tested with Ritalin, caffeine , and a placebo and had been rated daily by two caseworkers. In the behavioral areas of attentiveness and sociability and in anxiety and motor steadiness, Ritalin only equaled caffeine. As for side effects, caffeine had none, but Ritalin produced loss of appetite in three children and irritability in two.

The Garfield-Webster-Sloman study shows Ritalin and caffeine to possess in varying degree the ability to muffle the symptoms of the hyperactive child temporarily and superficially. Both leave untreated the underlying physiological and sometimes psychiatric disorders that are the source of the child's agitated and distraught condition. But for a few hours they can silence the signals of distress. What they do not share is a propensity for also creating immediately apparent, disagreeable side effects.

Of course, caffeine has its own ill effects. A single cup of coffee at breakfast and another at midday may not destroy appetite, cause weight loss, or produce nervousness or abdominal pain. Nevertheless, the beverage has long been recognized as posing threats, especially to young children. The pharmacological properties of caffeine are extensive. The drug's ability to stimulate the central nervous system extends to acting on the kidney to produce diuresis, quickening the heart muscle, relaxing the coronary arteries and bronchial tubes, and affecting the respiratory, vasomotor, and vagal centers in the medulla. It influences the heart myocardium, the blood vessels, the coronary circulation, the blood pressure, the gall bladder, the body's voluntary muscles, and the metabolism.[3]

A study at Boston University Medical Center surveyed 12,759 adult patients and found a strong correlation between coffee drinking and heart attacks. The results disclosed that if people drank one to five cups of coffee a day, their risk of having a heart attack was 60 per cent higher than that of persons who drank none. Another study reported bladder cancer risk to be 25 per cent higher in coffee drinkers (one or more cups a day) than in nondrinkers. Caffeine was the suspect because it has been shown to cause mutations of cells in tissue cultures.

Consumer Bulletin has warned that "coffee should not be used by cardiac, ulcer, or liver disease patients, by persons with high blood pressure or hyperthyroidism, nor by those who find that coffee gives them digestive discomfort or wakefulness." The same source stated that "coffee elevates the serum cholesterol level."[4] Other studies have indicated a link between coffee consumption and a low blood sugar level, as the caffeine can overstimulate the pancreas to produce too much insulin. These findings are drawn from the adult population, and what they reveal is doubly significant to the health of our children.

16
Megavitamins

Ella O., seven years and three months old, was a family referral, brought in by her foster parents because of her hyperactivity, temper tantrums, and school difficulties. Nothing was known of the child's natural parents other than that they were a couple in their twenties. Ella had been adopted at age one week.

The foster parents, who appeared to be reliable informants, said that Ella had first demonstrated problems when she entered a preschool in another state. There her behavior included random moving about, terrorizing the other children, and an inability to follow directions or pursue a task. Ella was asked to leave that school, and a year later she started kindergarten. Again she had trouble staying in one place, but she modified her attitude toward other children, was more acceptable, and completed one year. In the first grade her behavior excited little criticism, and to some extent she improved her schoolwork.

The family moved to Southern California, where Ella entered the second grade. At this time she had some problems with handwriting, showing occasional reversals such as "hg" for "gh." She was now reading at the fourth-grade level , high for her age, and yet it seemed she couldn't follow directions, as in art projects and mathematics.

Mrs. O. described Ella's temper tantrums as occurring usually in association with the increased pressures felt in getting ready for school or in going to bed promptly at half past eight. Her outbursts were accompanied by weeping and uncontrolled shouting. The foster mother denied that Ella exhibited any symptoms that might suggest convulsive seizures in connection with the tantrums. The foster parents had been told, by a relative who was a social worker, that Ella's behavior at home was caused by wanting to be the one in control and that adequate treatment would involve hospitalization.

Mrs. O. stated that the child was weighed once a week and that there had been a recent weight gain. She said that Ella had always had a very good appetite and had been free from excessive thirst, going to the bathroom at night, itching, and urinary tract or vaginal infections. Prenatal and perinatal records of course were not available. The baby had been bottle-fed. It was uncertain when she first sat up, stood, walked, or chose between left- and right-handedness. It was uncertain when she spoke her first words. Ella's foster mother explained that she had written down details of this kind in a baby book, but the volume along with a boxful of snapshots had somehow got lost in the move. She was positive that Ella had been toilet-trained at age two and had started preschool at three years.

The girl had received the usual inoculations and had contracted none of the common childhood diseases. Mrs. O. believed that this was due to a regimen that included multiple vitamins, B-complex, A, and D as well as E supplements and cod liver oil daily. Although Ella was free from liver, kidney, and bone or joint diseases, tuberculosis, venereal disease, diabetes, high blood pressure, and seizures or convulsions, she had had a heart murmur detected. Also, she had been the subject of a psychiatric evaluation and was in ongoing therapy.

As for the girl's social history, review of systems, general physical examination, mental status, cranial nerves, and associated neurophysiologic data, all were essentially noncontributory to the search for the cause or causes underlying this child's hyperactivity.

But associated biochemical data disclosed a high total bilirubin count in the blood. Bilirubin is a byproduct derived from the destruction of red blood cells either naturally or through pathological processes. Likewise, biochemical data revealed an excessively high assay of Vitamin A. The data recorded gamma globulin, an infection fighter in the blood serum, in low supply. All of this added up to an impression of possible Vitamin A toxicity, another impression of possible carbon monoxide chronic toxicity, and with the foregoing, a pathological child-parent relationship developing through the responses of a little girl in the grip of such toxicities.

In Ella's case history we see the influence of a well-intentioned, zealous, and somewhat overprotective foster mother who apparently was unaware that overdosages of vitamins may be toxic — particularly the fat soluble vitamins. The multiple vitamins coupled with additional cod liver oil would bring the Vitamin A into a toxic range. The treatment recommended was to discontinue the Vitamin A supplement dosage and to stress instead the treatment of the mixed dominance indicated in the child's writing reversals. Ella stabilized, and in several years went ahead to improve to the point of normalcy.

Persons who defend the use of stimulant drugs in the management of hyperactive children frequently cite as topmost authority the HEW panel that in January 1971 approved this practice, though only when the psychoactive medications were administered under medical supervision. But what is appropriate medical supervision? A popular assumption is that the family doctor assumes this supervisory role. However, many general practitioners have not been comfortable functioning in an area in which they have had little if any specialized training. More family doctors are likely to feel that way as the problems of malpractice insurance loom larger on their professional horizons and as the threat of legal action in defense of children's rights clouds the prescribing of drugs that can have harmful effects on children.

The HEW panel did note the basic issue involved in the problem of appropriate medical supervision:

> When available treatments cannot be confidently and appropriately delivered by physicians, they are perhaps best withheld until such treatments can be provided — especially with milder dysfunctions. This is not to say that severely afflicted hyperkinetic children should not or cannot receive available medical treatment. But until systems of continuing professional education and ready access to consultants are finished and perfected, some judgement about the pace at which unfamiliar treatments can be widely fostered is required. Finally, we must recognize that it is not only the scarcity of trained personnel, but factors such as poverty and inadequate educational facilities which prevent accessibility to individualized treatment.[1]

Poverty and educational shortcomings notwithstanding, it should be clear where the *medical* responsibility rests. But it is not really clear at all. U.S. medical schools have assigned the hyperactivity syndrome as a whole to their departments of psychiatry. Presumably they have done so because the surface manifestations of the hyperactivity disorder are related to behavior and learning disabilities. Hence most studies of the problem and recommendations of treatment have been made by psychiatrists. Unfortunately, psychiatrists today limit their effectiveness with patients by not paying attention to the patients' biological status before plunging ahead into the interpretation of esoteric symptoms. This explains the all-too-general willingness to drug a child into temporary states of passivity, receptivity, and compliance so that his or her psychological resources and processes may be examined and trained.

Those who believe that the pendulum has swung too far in the direction of psychotherapy — indeed, has not only swung but has stuck there — think that it is more than time to get back to medical science and to solve problems with scientific logic rather than post-Freudian theories. Among the spokesmen for such attitudes is Linus Carl Pauling, who has bluntly charged that psychiatry has failed.

But while Pauling as critic has focused attention on psychiatry's shortcomings, he has also complicated the problem by introducing an offshoot psychiatry of his own: orthomolecular psychiatry, a brainchild born late in its originator's career. Most people know Pauling as the advocate of megadoses of Vitamin C to prevent or cure the common cold.

The B-complex vitamins are water soluble, as is Vitamin C. Orthomolecular psychiatry as a dominant feature of therapy prescribes megadoses of the B-complex vitamin group for the treatment of mental illness, especially schizophrenia, and also in the treatment of alcoholism and mental disorders attributed to drug abuse. Here again Pauling has both admirers and critics. Many U.S. psychiatrists are highly critical. There are at least a handful, though, among orthomolecular psychiatry's converts who go further and advocate massive doses of the fat-soluble vitamins A, D, E, and K. These vitamins are not readily excreted, as water-soluble vitamins are believed to be, but are stored in the body. Very severe ill effects from both overdoses and deficiencies of fat-soluble vitamins are on medical record. A *deficiency* of Vitamin A can produce eye disorders that in the long run may result in blindness. Prolonged overdoses of the same vitamin can cause irritability, painful joints, thickening of bones, itching, thinning and drying of hair, retarded growth of children, symptoms resembling those of brain tumor, and even result in skin lesions with peeling of palms. There may be extraocular muscle paralysis. Overdoses of cod liver oil for a half-year period may result in vitaminosis A.[2]

Megavitamin dosages of Vitamin D above 150,000 units per day can be toxic. The symptoms may range through fatigue, lassitude, headache, depression, and psychosis to excessive thirst and urination. Four to six months on a regimen diet is required to clear the body of excess Vitamin D.[3]

Notwithstanding Vitamin B3's water solubility, a task force of the American Psychiatric Association has reported toxic reactions in patients arising from the prolonged megadosage administration of Vitamin B3. These included duodenal ulcer, abnormal liver function, hyperglycemia and extraordinary increases of serum uric acid.[4]

There can be little justification for using megavitamins to treat children who have been diagnosed as having "hyperactivity with minimal brain dysfunction" or "hyperkinesis with minimal learning disability" or some similarly described condition. This would be true even if the medication produced some improvement in the patient, for in that case it would be particularly important to learn why the child responded to the megavitamins. Yet, no simple, offhand answer to that question is sufficient; the effects of any one vitamin are too numerous.

Vitamin B_1 (thiamine) must be present for the biosynthesis of a coenzyme that in turn is essential to carbohydrate metabolism. Also, a child's good appetite, good intestinal functioning, and normally performing cardiovascular and nervous systems depend in part upon this vitamin. A condition known as Wernicke's encephalopathy, characterized by bleeding brain lesions, can develop as a result of thiamine deficiency following the intake of excessive amounts of alcohol or nutritional depletion. This vitamin deficiency may become a source of concern since, like drug addiction, adolescent alcoholism is widespread, especially among delinquent youth at all socioeconomic levels, while the nutritional deficiencies of junk foods consumed by children hardly require comment.

The Vitamin B complex includes a dozen factors, each one of which in its individual way, and some in a number of ways, is essential to health. Diseases of the skin and eyes are frequently seen in cases of Vitamin B complex insufficiency. A close relationship exists here since the skin, brain, nervous system and sense organs originate in the embryo ectoderm, so that physiologically the eyes may be described as the visible part of the brain.

Among the disorders that are related to flaws or the faulty functioning of B-complex vitamins, or that respond to its components, are pernicious anemia, beriberi, pellegra, inflammations, skin diseases, psychological disturbances, gastrointestinal ailments, dementia, and — as an outcome of some of these — death. Vitamins have essential roles in carbohydrate metabolism, blood clotting, the metabolism of amino acids, the manufacture of hemoglobin, the metabolism of fatty acids, of steroids, of phospholipids, and of heme. They are needed for respiration, digestion, and reproduction. They function independently and cooperatively.

But the human body is not made up of row upon row of test tubes in which chemical components are fuming away in their varied, independent reactions. Body and mind are not separate entities. Autism in the young patient may be owing to a toxicity, as in lead poisoning. It may be related to seizures or to trauma or to thyroid disturbance. The thyroid function is part of the endocrine system, as are the parathyroid glands, and therefore has a role in the regulation of the calcium and the phosphorus metabolism. In the pancreas, the endocrine system is represented by the islets of Langerhans, which regulate the flow of insulin and so control the level of blood sugar.

Good health is not maintained by bombarding the human body with megadoses of vitamins. This point is being pressed by Dr. Victor Herbert, vice chairman of medicine at the State University of New York's Downstate Medical Center. In several West Coast interviews, Dr. Herbert has stressed that megadoses of vitamins are worthless as therapy and, indeed, can in some cases be dangerous. He describes how vitamins unite with cell proteins, known as apoenzymes, to form a chemical group of holoenzymes and in this form stimulate normal body metabolism.

The apoenzyme content of the cell is limited, Dr. Herbert explains, and any vitamin taken in excess of the apoenzyme limit, the water-soluble ones included, become circulating chemicals whose activity may do harm to body processes.

According to Dr. Herbert, the foregoing is especially true of megadoses of Vitamins C and E. Among the ill effects of large doses of Vitamin C are a swelling and bleeding of the gums, a loosening of the teeth, muscular pain, skin roughening, adverse effects on growing bone, inaccurate outcomes of blood sugar level tests that present the peril of dangerously wrong doses of insulin being prescribed, falsely negative blood stool tests of patients being evaluated for intestinal bleeding, as well as inducing menstrual bleeding in pregnant women and possible destruction of substantial amounts of B_{12} ingested with food.

Herbert attributes to megadoses of Vitamin E such side effects as low blood sugar, intestinal disturbances, increased bleeding tendency, inflammation of the mouth and chapping of the lips, blurred vision, giddiness, fatigue, nausea, headaches, and decreased function of the male and female gonads.

Some of the effects described by this highly experienced clinical nutritionist run directly counter to the claims advanced by megavitamin enthusiasts. "I respect Linus Pauling," Dr. Herbert said in a newspaper interview, "but he's doing harm."[5]

Treatment with vitamins, as with any therapy or regimen, should not precede diagnosis. A comprehensive differential diagnosis should be the first step, and it should be performed by a physician who has in mind the entire patient rather than by one who thinks and prescribes in terms of the particular potential of a special medication or program of exercises, diet, or dietary supplement.

This applies with special emphasis and urgency to the treatment of hyperactive children. The victims of the syndrome have already spent far too much time in the no-man's-land between general medicine and psychiatry. Both specialties rely on stimulant drugs and both fail these children. Orthomolecular psychiatry with its copious floods of vitamins will not cure them either.

17
Lithium

THE DRUG LITHIUM, some of whose properties were possibly known 1500 years ago, has recently been considered as a medication for hyperactive children. The incentive for hoping that such treatment might succeed was found in the results obtained when lithium carbonate was used in the management of manic-depressive adults.

Manic-depression is a multiphasic disorder. In the manic phase, patients ride "highs" of sometimes wild exhilaration. Writers and artists have been known to reach creative pinnacles during a manic period. But the manic individual may also throw away a fortune, a career, or a marriage as he or she plunges along this phase's reckless, erratic, harebrained course. Mania may be chronic or, if the patient has intervals of normality, be termed recurrent. Dr. Mogens Schou, a Danish biochemist and psychiatrist, and others were reporting remarkable normalizing effects from administering lithium to manic patients during the early 1960s.[1]

The depressive phase in manic-depression is one of profound melancholia, despair, and suicidal impulses. Some patients alternate between highs and lows, but manic-depression's depressive phase is seen ten times as often as its manic. How much help lithium might give to depressive-phase patients remains uncertain; various antidepression drugs are believed to be more effective in treating depression.

Of particular interest, vis-à-vis hyperactivity in children, are two emerging conclusions: So-called alternating-phase manic-depressive illness has responded better to lithium than does recurrent depression alone; and Dr. Ronald R. Fieve and his colleagues at New York State Psychiatric Institute have seen value in a combination of lithium and antidepressant drugs.[2]

But are children ever manic-depressive? On this question psychiatrists do not agree. Might lithium be useful in treating a child who could possibly be diagnosed as being either "hyperactive" or "hypomanic," that is, suffering a mild manic disorder?

Across the Atlantic, two authorities seem to have replied in the affirmative to both questions. Dr. Anna-Lisa Annell, head of the department of child and youth psychiatry at Sweden's University of Uppsala and chief of the university's 35-bed children's psychiatric clinic, tried lithium over a four-year period with 60 children ranging in age from six to eighteen years. In half of the cases, the drug was ineffective. In the remaining half, it was useful therapeutically in preventing "highs," but less effective with depression.[3]

Dr. Eva A. Frommer, in charge of the children's psychiatric clinic at St. Thomas's Hospital, London, is quoted as believing that doctors generally fail to diagnose depression in children because "suffering in childhood tends to be ignored by a society which deludes itself that childhood is the halcyon period of life, and fails to take the reality experienced by the child seriously."[4]

A Canadian correspondent addresses the same subject in a letter to a medical journal:

> It was many years ago that the late D. W. Winnicott discussed the frequency of manic or hypomanic activity as a defense against depression in children.
>
> The constant, restless, seemingly purposeless activity, the impulsiveness, the reduced attention span, the emotional immaturity and irritability, and the poor judgment which you describe as part of the picture of the hyperactive child are part of the picture of mania at any age . . . These symptoms may be due to many causes; surely by now we should all be alert to the possibility that one of these causes is a defense against depression. The presence of more or less conscious wondering whether one should give in to depression or "fight it off" by overactivity and cheerfulness is not confined to adults.

When manic excitement is considered as a possibility, then in interviewing the child one is much more apt to take a history which will include the possibility of the child being chronically depressed. In the simplest examples the child may be surprisingly ready to discuss depression and the causes of his sadness, and may even begin to talk about the relationship of his overactivity to his hopes of avoiding its becoming apparent in himself to others.[5]

It may be relevant to mention here that some psychiatrists believe that an obsessive-compulsive reaction is actually a depression in disguise.[6] Reference also should be made to Dr. Frommer's use of lithium for emotionally disturbed children: "Among them were children who showed behavior which, in an adult, would suggest a diagnosis of hypomania: Their play was restless and aimless, their conversation disjointed, their ability to concentrate so poor they were virtually unteachable. [In the United States, who can doubt that similar behavior would be construed as evidence of childhood hyperactivity?] In some of these cases, the symptoms subsided on lithium therapy. Certain other children, described as periodically falling into moods marked by depressive features (that is, somatic complaints) and temper outbursts of dreadful proportions, were helped when lithium was added to their antidepressant drug therapy." Dr. Frommer reported that lithium treatment needed close supervision because it occasionally led to or contributed to a depression. Yet the lithium-antidepressant combination succeeded so well that children in several cases asked to continue on the medication until they "felt really well again."[7]

It should be noted that lithium did not cure but merely controlled or subdued the behavior of hyperactive (or, questionably, hypomanic) children. Lithium's role was like that of Ritalin or one of the amphetamines, which also fall short of achieving complete response in any group of children.

Could lithium carbonate be effective in those cases in which Ritalin, Thorazine, Benadryl, and Dilantin have failed?

Dr. Lawrence L. Greenhill, Dr. Ronald O. Rieder, Dr. Paul H. Wender, Dr. Monte Buchsbaum, and Dr. Theodore P. Zahn, undertook to find out. They had reviewed the studies reported by Dyson, Annell, Frommer, and Rikin, each of which had found lithium effective in an area of hyperactive, psychotic, hypomanic, depressed, or emotional instability.

Nine children, aged six to sixteen, were selected on the basis of hyperactivity, nonresponsiveness to stimulant drugs, school difficulties, refractoriness to psychotherapy, and freedom from psychosis, kidney, liver, heart, or thyroid diseases. The procedures followed in this investigation give the impression of thorough preparation, precaution, baseline evaluative measures, neuropsychiatric examination, testing methods continuing, and post-study observations. The outcome found lithium carbonate "a poor drug for the treatment of intractible hyperactivity." (This study was of course *planned* to test lithium's effectiveness on hyperactive children who did *not* respond to stimulant medication.[8])

Lithium has toxic possibilities and can even be fatally toxic. The use of lithium chloride as a dietary, sodium-free table salt was an agent in widely publicized poisonings and a factor in three deaths in 1949.

Lithium carbonate medication, given orally, is effective because of the action of the lithium ions, which alter the transport of sodium ions in the body and nerve cells. Lithium reacts in some manner with one of the most subtle and mysterious functionings of the autonomic nervous system. The thyroid gland becomes host to strong concentrations of lithium ions, which are also found in muscle, bone, the kidney, liver, cerebrospinal fluid, brain, and of course in blood plasma.

Lithium appears to be somewhat better suited to the hospital environment than to the world outside, inasmuch as frequent blood samplings may be required for making the ion counts to determine the body's content of the drug. Toxic accumulations of lithium in the patient must be avoided, and great care must be taken when the medication is given to persons with heart or kidney problems.

Lithium therapy has side effects. The early ones include nausea, vomiting, diarrhea, stomach pain, muscular weakness, thirst, urinary frequency, a dazed, tired, sleepy feeling, and a hand tremor, which remains as a long-term side effect. Abnormally excessive thirst and urination are later side effects. Weight gain is a problem. Thyroid reactions can occur and a possibility of goiter development exists, especially in patients with pre-existing defects of thyroid functioning.

Other side effects — and sidelights — accompanied or followed lithium's appearance as a sophisticated element in the medical scene.

In the year that lithium became available to the University of Rochester, New York, the number of manic-phase patients zoomed from the usual eight or nine admissions to fifty. Dr. Aaron Satloff, who obtained the FDA's permission to use the drug, believes that admissions swelled because doctors wanted their patients to have the new therapy.

Could it be that hyperactivity similarly ballooned into high visibility when it was believed that something could be done for the hyperactive child?

At the same time, the advent of lithium focused attention on a diagnostic problem. Lithium is helpful to the manic patient, but not to the schizo-affective patient. Dr. Satloff and Dr. David Tinling were face to face with the difficulty of differentiating between manic-phase and schizo-affective patients. Until then, mania had been diagnosed chiefly by excluding a diagnosis of schizophrenia. Also, they began to look sharply at the criteria for the diagnosis of schizophrenia used by psychiatrists of different theoretical orientations.[9]

But just as it became more important to differentiate between varieties of mental illness, it becomes more urgent also to distinguish between the variety of causes and their symptomatic evidences within the hyperactivity syndrome. Is the hyperactive child's problem one of hypomania? Or depression disguised as hypomania? Or is the problem physiological, and sometimes as simple as pinworms? Should the treatment be lithium or psychoanalysis or a vermifuge? These are questions that can only, in the child's best interests, be answered on the basis of adequate individual diagnosis.

18

Brain Surgery:
The Irreversible Treatment

SUGGESTED TREATMENTS FOR HYPERACTIVITY vary widely but do have some features in common. Almost all are founded on the belief that hyperactivity is "one disease, having one cause and one cure" — each of these treatments, of course, offering that one cure.

The proferred therapies range from the relatively benign two cups of coffee daily to the irreparable damage wrought by destructive neurosurgical procedures. Lobotomy, the cutting of nerve pathways on the frontal lobes of the brain, was first performed by Dr. Egas Moniz. He drilled holes through the skull and used a leucotome technique to cut through the nerve fibers that connect the brain's frontal lobes with its lower brain centers. The operation was then known as "prefrontal lobotomy" or "prefrontal leucotomy." Later, the surgical instruments were inserted into the brain, through the eye orifices above the eyeballs.

In recent years a kind of neurosurgery and thalamotomy has focused on areas of the thalamus. Located in the lower brain, the thalamus is an egg-sized relaying station that forwards sensory information to the cerebrum above and also serves as a reacting center where incoming sense-gathered stimuli are translated into physical responses, emotional reactions, or both. In this modern neurosurgery, holes are again drilled in the skull, but on its side, and the cutting instruments may be replaced by electrodes, which burn away the brain tissue.[1]

Lobotomy in Dr. Moniz's day was rather naively greeted with enthusiasm as offering a swift and indisputable victory over some severe pathophysiological and psychiatric disorders. The patients were psychotic, and their behavioral symptoms had not improved under other modalities of treatment. After twenty years, during which thousands of lobotomies were performed, it was recognized that, in the roughly 50 per cent of these operations that could be termed successful, the improvement was only temporary. Some patients behaved worse than before, and some were reduced to the status of human vegetables.

The Board of Directors of the National Association for Mental Health (NAMH) adopted a position statement on June 5, 1973. It declared that psychosurgery should not be used except when the patient is in such great personal distress due to his mental disorder that he or she, by free choice, would prefer surgery rather than the existing condition. The procedure to be followed should receive the written approval of at least two other neurosurgeons not associated in practice with the surgeon selected to perform the surgery. The patient should have legal representation present when any final decision is made regarding the operation to make certain the patient fully understands the decision and knows that he or she can refuse to go through with it even if he or she may have previously agreed to it.

"Psychosurgery," as defined by the NAMH, means "surgical procedures on the structurally intact brain to produce behavioral change, not to correct or eradicate organic pathology." The NAMH position statement was prepared partly as a response to "those who are seriously and properly concerned about the possibility that psychosurgery will be practiced unethically and experimentally upon hospitalized patients, members of minority groups, and others unable to protect themselves, or that it may not be used as a treatment procedure to correct a specific disorder but as a means to alter or control persons who act aggressively in social struggles for the recognition of their rights."

Would the "others unable to protect themselves" include children? Certainly children confronted by the threat of brain surgery to "modify" their behavior have no choice in the matter; the decision must in their case be made by the parent(s), legal guardian, or public institution.

On the record, both in this country and abroad, children have been the victims of surgery that destroys brain areas. Phyllis Breggin, writing in *Mental Hygiene*, believes it may be happening at the present time: "The press and the Project to Examine Psychiatric Technology have uncovered many psychosurgeons who were operating and not publishing the results. Just as the number of doctors who prescribe amphetamines for hyperactive children is unknown, so the psychosurgeons may go about their operations unrestrained by review boards or even a central reporting system . . ."[2] This observer calls attention to an Indian neurosurgeon who practices "sedative surgery" on children to correct such symptoms as "wandering tendency" and "restlessness." Another practitioner cited is a Japanese neurosurgeon who has reported hypothalamotomies on 79 patients, characterized as "violent, aggressive, and restless," of whom 26 were under age fifteen. Two prominent neurosurgeons in the United States reported frontal lobotomies on a dozen children, aged from four to fourteen, with results described as "unsatisfactory in some ways, since none of these children ever returned to normal home living, but satisfactory in others, since they were less aggressive in the hospital after the operations."[3] This may call to mind treatment resulting in deaths of patients in California state mental hospitals during the 1970s.

It is quite possible to see parallels between psychosurgery and the administering of psychoactive drugs. Some children do not respond to stimulant drugs in their prescribed dosages. A few parents then seek to increase the dosages — and have succeeded, as we know from Dr. Gerald Solomons's study of this problem. But increased dosages are not always the answer. We should be alert to the possibility of a parent, who himself or herself could be on the verge of collapsing into a mental and physical breakdown, seeking psychosurgery as a means of subduing an extremely hyperactive child. Remember that the damage incurred through brain surgery is for life, and in our rapidly moving age of medical research, a child's problem may be solved next month, next year, or perhaps three years hence.

We can put a man on the moon and a robot on Mars; surely we ought to be able to control hyperactivity in our children. This attitude implies that landings in space are complex and difficult achievements, compared to which straightening out our children should be a simple matter. The concept goes far to explain the instant, eager acceptance that is awarded to any new treatment, whether by pill, allergy-related diet, or megavitamin attack in force.

The human mind is more complex and miraculous than all its works put together. We should not be surprised that our brain, our central and autonomic nervous systems, the organs and the metabolisms and biochemical processes, are liable to profound and baffling disorders. The hyperactivity and learning disability of a child constitute a syndrome that is in itself a complicated symptom. It is not to be laid to rest by the psychosurgical crippling of the child's brain.

PART IV

NEUROPSYCHIATRIC DIAGNOSIS: WHAT HOPE IS THERE AHEAD?

19
Warren M.: A Workup of a Hyperactive Patient

WARREN M., AT AGE TEN YEARS and three months, came to the Southern California Neuropsychiatric Institute on the referral of a physician practicing in a rural, citrus and avocado district. This doctor described the boy as handicapped by severe learning difficulties and by impulsive, restless, inattentive, purposeless behavior, both the learning difficulties and the behavior being of the kind characteristic of hyperactive children.

The report that accompanied the referral further described Warren as having a breathing problem and as having experienced episodes of partial hearing loss during periods of recurring earache. In addition, the young patient had a history of heart murmur; however, he had recently been studied with chest films and an EKG by a cardiologist, who declared the condition to be benign.

Warren's parents requested an appointment for five weeks distant, to coincide with an agricultural seminar that Mr. M., an avocado grower, planned to attend. The period was one of gasoline shortages, and he could drive by way of La Jolla, leaving his wife and son at the institute's door.

At first glance, the youngster who entered my consulting room with his mother appeared to be of average sturdy build and seemed normal for his age. He was blond and blue-eyed. But in contrast to Mrs. M.'s rosy complexion, Warren had the drained look sometimes seen in patients who have been unable to throw off the effects of a past illness. In hyperactive children, such a drained look may be linked to some existing, underlying physiological disorder. It is likely to be a serious disorder, yet one that is expressed only through central nervous system irritability.

In these cases, all that parents and teachers can see are the outward signs — or signals — displayed in the hyperactive child's behavior and school failure. The hidden cause may perhaps be a toxic condition. (Very recent studies strongly point to lead poisoning as one among the significant causes of hyperactivity. See Chapter 6.) However, hyperactivity presenting very much the same surface symptoms may be traced to metabolic, postinfectious, structural, or some other cause among the many often-implicated disorders and deficiencies.

Warren had indeed been referred because of his "hyperactivity," "learning difficulties," and "impulsive, restless, inattentive, purposeless behavior." Yet these and equivalent terms, even when employed by physicians, serve only to label the patient with tags descriptive of his or her symptoms. The labels are not useful in defining medically the nature of an individual child's problem — its cause, its probable future course and outcome, or its appropriate treatment. The labels tell us nothing about the forces that are at work — or, it would be better to say, are not at work but at war — racketing and rampaging about in raging, destructive, ungovernable ways.

In order to help these children, it is necessary to explore first their hidden malfunctionings and to determine what treatment will halt and heal the strife within each individual. In each case, therapy must be preceded by a process of differential diagnosis.

Neuropsychiatric diagnosis is a development of modern, advanced differential investigation, well suited to the study of the hyperactive child. It is especially wide in its scope, taking into account the ills of both body and mind in an integrated medical exploration that uses the resources and insights of physiological, biochemical, neurological and psychiatric science in a single, coordinated assessment of the patient's status. It diagnoses the whole person; it does not see the individual as merely the host to some one ailment. Neuropsychiatric diagnosis is especially deep-seeking in its far-ranging and exhaustive searches; and it is especially sophisticated in its scientific tools and their use. It is also particularly tenacious in pursuing any detail that may possibly contribute to solving a patient's problem.

The very first rule in neuropsychiatric diagnosis is that subtle dysfunction requires subtle, meticulous techniques to arrive at an accurate evaluation.

"You see," I said in explaining to Mrs. M. why Warren's diagnosis would consume all of two office days and part of a third, "nothing can be overlooked, and nothing can be taken for granted."

Warren would shortly be excused to be weighed and measured, getting him started on a careful, comprehensive general physical examination. She and I would then have a chance to discuss sensitive material alone. Meanwhile, I began our interview with inquiries to draw out and formulate the boy's history through reviewing his symptoms as they had appeared. How and when had she first noticed that her son was distractible?

"Why, I think it really started after we moved into the new house." Mrs. M. explained that when Warren was six, the family's home on the avocado ranch had burned to the ground. Thereafter the family occupied rental quarters in town until, two and a half years later, a new ranch house was built and furnished.

When Warren had left the room with a staff member, his mother spoke more explicitly. "Doctor" — she spread open her hands, palms up — "I just can't understand my own child. He was a fussy baby to begin with. After that, he was a tense, nervous little child. I used to think it was because he was our 'only,' and because his health wasn't the best. He had one case of sniffles after another. But when we moved into town, it seemed to me he picked up physically and showed he could make good adjustments, too. I can't remember that he ever balked at going to school. He brought home good report cards. He never had any trouble with his teachers. Now he's in trouble all the time."

I asked precisely what was happening.

"He's in squabbles and scraps with kids who used to be his good friends. He pesters his teacher. And he isn't learning anything in school. He's even backsliding. His handwriting and his spelling were better last year than they are now."

I sought more specific data. "Can you think back to a particular incident? Did anything happen that might have been instrumental in bringing about this change?"

"Doctor, it's the same school. The school hasn't changed. The other children haven't changed. It's just Warren." Suddenly Mrs. M. looked thoughtful.

"There's one difference. Warren takes the school bus now. Right at the start, too, he complained because the driver made him sit way at the back of the bus where some big kids picked on him — well, they teased him. He wanted permission to sit up front next to a boy of his own age."

Warren's parents had observed that the bus was still nearly empty when Warren boarded it. One morning, Mr. M. waited at the roadside stop to ask the driver to let Warren sit up front. The driver explained that he had the first children go to the back seats so late-comers would not be crowding and tripping over each other in the aisle trying to find places. If he made an exception for Warren, he said he would have to let all the other children choose their seats and seatmates. He was not about to risk starting up and shifting gears in the old, jerky bus while kids with armloads of books were on their feet and moving around. If he did, somebody's child would get hurt badly someday. Besides, he had a schedule to keep.

"The man was probably right," Warren's mother said. "We didn't take it up with the principal or the school board. My husband doesn't really believe in parents fighting their kids' battles for them, anyway."

I asked how Warren had reacted to the disappointment.

"He cried. And he wet his bed for the first time since he was five."

Asked when it was that she first thought of her son as "hyperactive," Mrs. M. replied that it was after hearing his grade school teacher apply the word to Warren. This teacher considered him to be the least troublesome of four hyperactive boys in her classroom. He wasn't destructive or insolent or rebellious. But it seemed to her that a hundred times a day Warren's hand was raised, fingers sometimes urgently snapping, to plead for her attention and help. He sought assistance with dividing 9 into 72, although he had earlier learned the multiplication tables. He wanted permission to sharpen a pencil; if he had been free to move about the room at will, she believed he would have used the sharpener dozens of times daily. Repeatedly he asked to leave to get a drink at the fountain in the corridor. He always seemed thirsty. He would forget his study assignments. Reminded, he sat squirming behind an open book, grinding his teeth with a nervous insistence that drove the teacher up the wall.

"I know the feeling," Mrs. M. said. "He has another trick of taking a big, gasping breath and then closing his mouth and holding his nose while he blows hard to 'pop' his ears. He says he hears better after he does that. To me, it's more irritating than the teeth grinding."

I asked what steps the teacher had taken or suggested be taken in managing Warren.

"She recommended that we ask a doctor to prescribe Ritalin to calm him. We thought, well, if it would do any good . . . But it didn't."

In opening the physiological examination phase of the interview, my first questions were aimed at getting a picture of Warren's twenty-four-hour day. His mother said he was supposed to be in bed by eight to eight thirty, but often he retired reluctantly. He slept with one pillow. (This point was raised with reference to his breathing and possible heart complications.) Warren's sleep was restless, marred by nightmares and, recently, by bedwetting when he was especially fatigued and out of sorts after a bad day. He was called at seven in the morning, and usually did not appear refreshed.

Warren drank several cups of cocoa at breakfast. He would eat a large bowl of dry cereal (a brand with an exceptionally high sugar content) or a cooked cereal with a generous sprinkling of sugar. His favorite box lunch included a thermos bottle of cocoa, a peanut butter and jelly sandwich, and an apple or orange. He ate an afterschool snack of milk and cookies. The family's evening meal was consistently meat and vegetables with a green or a fruit salad. The boy's thirst and his craving for sweets might have suggested blood sugar difficulties. However, his mother had never observed that he perspired after the main meal nor had she detected other indications of insulin-sugar-ratio imbalance. We, of course, would give Warren a five-hour glucose tolerance test to check this.

Mrs. M. believed her son preferred watching television to playing outdoors. She would turn off the set to stop his nervous grinding of teeth or ear popping while viewing TV. He did enjoy a game of Chinese checkers with his father.

Many inquiries in the course of a comprehensive interview with a parent are fruitless. Nevertheless, the questions must be asked in every case. I probed further concerning headaches, toothaches, and stomachaches. Warren's mother was asked to search her memory for any episodes of vomiting, dizziness, indigestion, or diarrhea that, even though she might not be aware of their cause, could be significant in the light of the total neuropsychiatric evaluation.

The development history of a human being begins with the months before birth. It is a period that poses the possibility of complications that can have the severest consequences. During pregnancy, Mrs. M. had gained more than 40 pounds. She had also suffered a kidney infection accompanied by sugar in her urine. Warren's birth was by Caesarean section, and his mother related that there had been delay with the newborn infant's breathing. "I can worry myself sick," she said, "when I think that all his troubles really began then and there, and I don't know if they can ever really be cured."

I pointed out that Warren's handicaps at birth, if any, had not barred him from doing well during his first school years.

"Yes, that's true," she said, brightening a little.

"Besides, hyperactivity is hardly ever hopeless if a diligent effort is made to get to the real roots of a youngster's trouble."

I quoted the second rule of neuropsychiatric diagnosis: The search cannot be directed solely to any one suspected cause, no matter how probable that one may appear to be and even though it is the only cause visibly present.

Too frequently there are lurking problems in other areas — infections, diseases, nervous disorders, allergies, tumors, organic dysfunctions, or it may be some deficiency among the many hormones that are essential to a healthily functioning body. Such a single, overlooked complication can totally defeat a course of treatment that would otherwise effectuate a cure.

We resumed Warren's developmental history. When did he first sit up, stand, speak, walk, and respond to toilet training? Warren had reached these milepost "firsts" at ages ranging from the normal to the slow normal, as measured by the usually accepted standards. His mother did not recall that as a baby he ever engaged in head banging or body rocking in the crib.

The boy's medical history included inoculations for polio (three times), diphtheria, measles, and a tetanus shot. He had received medical attention following a nonpoisonous snakebite. His childhood illnesses were mumps, bronchitis, and numerous colds and sore throats, which sometimes were associated with earaches and poor hearing. On one occasion he was diagnosed as having hives after he and a neighbor gorged on new-crop tangerines picked from the neighbor's tree. He was extremely sensitive to smoke.

The family medical history can be valuable in suggesting genetic links underlying health problems. Warren's mother knew that two of her aunts had kidney disorders similar to her own. In her husband's family were instances of gall bladder problems, stomach ulcers, and colitis. She was not aware of heart and lung symptoms or of allergies among either her own or her husband's relatives.

It is important to know what drugs have been taken by a hyperactive child. In recent years, pharmaceutical products have become more and more specialized and potent and, by the same token, more and more profound in their effects upon living organisms. Miracles of healing have been achieved through their use. Disasters have followed their misuse. Well-documented charges have been made that the FDA has given its stamp of approval to new medications without adequately researching their dangers (see Chapter 2).

A careful diagnostician is interested in what medications are being taken by other members of the young patient's family — this in part because drugs are not always kept out of the reach of curious small children. Then, too, a discussion of prescribed medicines may awaken a parent's recollection of some illness or injury. In Warren's case, questioning at this stage elicited the information that the boy had been taken off Ritalin because the stimulant drug caused an excessively rapid heartbeat.

We moved on to the youngster's social history, and the focus turned to how Warren's environment and activities might relate to his hyperactivity. I inquired about pets in the home. Birds and animals, especially as they grow old or are ill, are possible sources of parasitic infections. Warren did have a dog, described by Mrs. M. as short-haired, young, and healthy. The dog was allowed in the house but not permitted to sleep in Warren's bedroom. The cats on the ranch were not house pets; they were hunters who kept down the gopher population in the avocado grove.

The house was heated by an oil furnace with forced-air circulation. A wood-burning fireplace in the family room had been converted to electric because of Warren's sensitivity to smoke. Warren did not have hobbies that would place him in contact with toxic glues and dangerous chemicals. He had never displayed cravings for unnatural foods and had not been observed biting or chewing on twigs, sticks, leaves, and the like, any of which might be poisonous or have been sprayed with pesticide. Mr. M.'s agricultural fertilizers and spraying materials were stored in a padlocked shed.

The interview ended with a review of systems; that is, a review of all complaints of the patient's head, eyes, ears, nose, throat, chest, abdomen, general urinary tract, and extremities. It comes before the general physical examination, and it may provide clues that should be especially pursued during that examination.

"Regarding Warren's head, has there been any record of seizures? Or a head injury? A loss of consciousness? Has he ever been in an automobile accident? Do you know of his ever falling from a tree or from playground equipment, or has he ever taken a bad skateboard tumble? Has he ever complained of headaches? Where did he say it hurt? What kind of pain did he complain of? Dull? Throbbing?"

My other questions were directed to the possibility of Warren having been troubled by blurred or double vision. Had he ever mentioned seeing rings around lights? Had she ever noticed that her son sometimes seemed not to see objects that were in his normal field of vision?

Mrs. M. replied "No, Doctor" and "Hardly ever" to most of these and similar queries.

The genito-urinary tract review suggested that Warren's bedwetting, occurring more frequently toward the end of the school week, was associated with fatigue and emotional disturbance. His mother did not recall abdominal symptoms such as diarrhea, constipation, nausea, vomiting, and black or bloody stools. She had never noticed impairments of movement in the boy's use of his limbs, hands, and feet, or his having cramps or weakness in his extremities. She stated that his skin tanned in a normal, healthy fashion. She remembered diaper rash during infancy, and a later instance of ringworm.

Finally, in the endocrine-metabolic investigation, Mrs. M. believed that her son was unusually affected by extremes of heat and cold. He seemed "listless and headachy" during the Southern California so-called Santa Ana heat spells, but she also thought that at these times he was weakened by gratifying his excessive thirst. She recognized that his craving for sweets was excessive, but at the same time she felt he needed the quick energy supplied by sugar in his diet. In conclusion, Mrs. M. expressed a fear that her son was "gradually losing ground" and was "being worn down by his hyperactivity thing."

Impressions gained during the initial interview of a neuropsychiatric diagnosis are, of course, tentative. While it is true that the patient (or the patient's parent or foster parent) will "tell the doctor the diagnosis," it is also true that parents differ vastly in their skill as observers and their ability to communicate, just as physicians differ in their skill as listeners and their ability to understand lucidly what may be said falteringly and ambiguously. Patients and the parents of patients may tell the physician not only the diagnosis but a great deal else that is trivial or is critical of the child's teacher or is merely repetitious.

Particularly in diagnosing children, the general physical examination marks a dramatic change in the neuropsychiatric evaluation procedures. Up to this point, the focus has been on the past symptoms and past treatment of the patient. The general physical and neurological examinations look to the child's present status and bring the examining physician into immediate contact with the evidence of well-being and of ailment, of the normal and the abnormal. These are examinations of critical importance, and yet too often they are indifferently performed.

There is an opportunity here for the physician to put the young patient at ease by conducting the examination gently enough to allay a youngster's apprehensions yet firmly enough to gain the child's confidence. I began by taking Warren's hands in my own, turning them this way and that, flexing his fingers, turning his palms, and scanning his nails. Fingernails, by their ridging and other structural peculiarities, may betray metabolic problems. Warren's nails were normal in appearance, his skin in healthy condition, and the range of movement in his hands and arms was satisfactory.

I found the boy to be in the upper third percentile for height in his age and sex group. He was in the 50th percentile for weight, and in the upper third percentile for head size. His blood pressure on both the right and the left side was normal. His pulse was 60 and his vision 20–20.

There followed in quick succession a series of tests to determine whether his cranial nerves were intact. The olfactory nerve responded to an aromatic (cloves). Field of vision for the left and the right eye was ascertained to be normal. With an ophthalmoscope, the interior of each eye was studied, with satisfactory results that would later be confirmed by fundus photography.

Throughout the examination, Warren betrayed scarcely a trace of the hyperactivity that so distressed his teachers and troubled his parents. He submitted to a rather threatening bimanual visual stimuli technique for checking occipital integrity; that is, checking the functioning of the area of the brain where images arriving from the two eyes are blended into a single image. He did not flinch when his pupils were examined with a tiny, brilliant light beam. He did not startle when his reaction to very near optical stimulus was observed. Soon thereafter, his nerves were being examined for their reactions to pinpricks. Some of the tests required adequate responses. Other responses, such as the "snout," "grasp," and "suck," had they occurred, would have evidenced developmental regression, for these are normally found only at the infantile level.

Warren's restraint during the neurological examination did not prove that he would be capable of equally calm behavior in different circumstances. Quite possibly his interest was captured by the novelty of his surroundings. It is very likely that he responded to the element of challenge in the examining techniques — when he was told to close his eyes first and then touch his finger to his nose, or when he was requested to walk barefooted in heel-and-toe manner across the room with his eyes shut, to stop, and to remain motionless in this "Romberg" position for at least 15 seconds. The boy's cooperative attitude can also be explained by referring to a number of educational experiments that tend to show that hyperactive children learn best in very small classes with one-to-one, teacher-to-pupil instruction. Surely there can scarcely be a more completely one-to-one working relationship than that which exists between patient and physician throughout a neurological examination.

Warren's acuity of hearing was determined by means of a watch ticking at a distance of 5 centimeters from each ear. His hearing was further examined in relation to bone conduction of sound. He gagged properly when his palate was tested and protruded his tongue on request.

Handedness (right, left, and mixed, ambidextrous or uncertain) correlates significantly with hyperactivity in children. The syndrome is found relatively more frequently in youngsters who are left-handed or have mixed dominance. The reason is ascribed to the crossing over of the motor nerve fibers in the human brainstem and spinal cord. Because of it, the right cerebral hemisphere controls the left side of the body, while the left half of the brain governs the right side. In this, the most specialized area of the brain, development most frequently favors right-handedness.

Warren was asked to look at a wall chart, using a toy telescope lying on a desk. He picked up the scope with his right hand and raised it to his right eye. He threw a ball with his right hand and kicked it with his right foot. He had no problems of mixed dominance. Aside from a minor irregularity detected during the eye examination, his physical and neurological findings were satisfactory.

Of course, none of this proved that the boy was not hyperactive or that he was capable of functioning normally in school. But neither did any of it point conclusively to why he was hyperactive.

Warren had already received a more comprehensive examination than is given to the great majority of children who are seen by physicians before being treated for hyperactivity with stimulant drugs or, less frequently, with tranquilizing medications. And this "majority" are but a small number of the many children whom the public schools consider hyperactive.*

---

*In Chicago, for example, of the thousands of children labeled hyperactive, 6100 identified as having learning disabilities were placed in special classrooms during the 1974–1975 school year, when they numbered approximately 1.5 per cent of the children in the city's elementary schools. Dr. Irving Abrams, medical director of the Chicago public schools, has stated that no one really knows how many of these youngsters are receiving medication. (*Clinical Psychiatry News*, May 1976, p. 44.)

My investigation of Warren's difficulties now moved on to the group of sophisticated procedures that provide associated neuropsychiatric data. As a matter of convenience, the funduscopic examination is completed in the laboratory setting. The "fundus," or base of each eye is recorded on color film through the use of specialized photographic equipment and techniques. As well as confirming earlier ophthalmoscopic findings, the funduscope films provide a permanent record to serve as a base for reference in the event of future papilledema (swelling), changes in the retinal blood vessels, and so forth. Such study of the fundus yielded the clue that directed suspicion to Debby B.'s underlying heart problem (see Chapter 5).

Incidentally, the stairs to the laboratory and its adjacent examining rooms give me a further opportunity to evaluate my young patient's mental and physical development as evidenced in his walking and climbing stairs. Significant clues are found in a child's manner of responding to the lab technician, especially in speech — his tone, vocabulary, and phrasing. In the light of what was known of Warren's home and social environment, his speech response was slightly lower than average quality.

Among the associated neurophysiologic procedures, the one most familiar to the public is the electroencephalograph, or EEG. An EEG provides an assessment of the brain's electrical activity. This is a relatively new diagnostic field, although the existence of the brain's electrical activity was demonstrated as early as 1929.

The EEG magnifies the impulses its electrodes receive from the brain and passes these along to a pen positioned over a sheet of paper. The magnified impulses guide the pen on the paper, and so create an encephalogram tracing as a record of the brain's waves. The tracing provides useful screening information.

However, the EEG is only one among other associated neurophysiologic data-gathering devices, though it is the only one mentioned as having been used in many of the hyperactivity studies reported in recent years by university medical school departments of psychiatry. That is unfortunate, for despite its specific usefulness the EEG has a limited reliability. There is not full agreement as to what constitutes a "normal tracing." If physicians get what they are satisfied to regard as normal tracings, they still cannot rule out the possibility that their patients may be victims of nonfunctional pathology. Furthermore, the EEG has been known to pick up electrical activities other than just those originating in the brain. Hypoxia (oxygen deficiency), metabolic rate, body temperature, emotional state, blood sugar and pH, changes in carbon dioxide tension, and water and electrolyte balance have all been cited as capable of altering the EEG record. Certainly the EEG does provide a record of the presence of tumors, hemorrhages, infections, deficiency states, and drug intoxication, but it does so in a nonspecific, indistinguishable manner.

The technician pasted a set of tiny electrodes to Warren's head at points selected as corresponding to areas of the brain within. For children, the process is wholly painless. (With adults, the electrodes are inserted under the scalp so that pinprick sensations are felt by the patient. The equally effective paste method takes longer.) The task of each electrode is to pick up the tiny impulses of electrical activity in its sector of the brain and to pass these impulses along to the recording mechanism. Thus, it is possible to identify the source of the wave activity within the brain.

When I came to study Warren's EEG, the tracing was abnormal as revealed by its dysrhythmic quality. But it lacked the focal characteristic, without which confidence in the EEG must be low. It testified that something of a pathophysiological nature troubled — indeed, tormented — the boy, but it did not specify what.

Occasionally hyperactivity has its origin in brain tumors, abscesses, or bleeding within the membranes that wrap the brain. Following the EEG, Warren was examined by echoencephalography, or SEG. Diagnosis is achieved by directing ultrasonic waves into the head, perpendicular to the skull, and picking up the midline echo on the right and left sides as registered by a transolucer. A disparity of more that 3 millimeters is considered a significant shift. A normal finding is expressed as "echo was midline." Warren's SEG found that "echo was midline." Had it been otherwise, the presence of some lesion in the brain might have been determined by a brain scan, perhaps by EMI C-A-T Scan. Both are techniques in which radioactive metals are intravenously injected. These accumulate in brain tumors, dead tissues, and other lesions, probably because blood-brain barrier disruption occurs in such affected areas. C-A-T is a density-sensitive method, with findings that are speeded by computer assistance.

It must be said that these ultrasophisticated diagnostic devices are appropriate for very few hyperactive children. Remember that the scanning procedures do not reach the whole host of metabolic, postinfectious, anemic, calcium-phosphate, and other problems. The resulting danger is that the failure of the scanning techniques to disclose an organic or structural flaw may lead to a too-hasty conclusion that the child's underlying problem must be psychiatric.

A very valuable technique is electronystagmography (ENG). As in an EEG, electrodes are used, but they are placed above, below, and at the sides of the eyes, the positioning dictated by their relationship to the eye pupils. Nystagmus, in pathology, means "a spasmodic, involuntary motion of the eyeball." The eyeballs are connected to the inner ear as well as to the cranial nerves that have to do with eye movements by means of a bundle of nerve fibers called the medial longitudinal fasciculus (MLF).

At issue in the ENG is an eye-ear relationship as the source of nystagmus. The inner ear houses the organs of equilibrium. As children know, it is not difficult to whirl around and around until dizziness ensues. This occurs because tiny, fluid-containing organs of the inner ear communicate to the brain our sensations of rising, falling, stooping, or jumping. When one stops spinning, the thickish fluid in the ear vessels does not instantly subside. Instead, the brain still receives inner ear signals indicating the body's continuing whirling movement. The landscape appears to wheel out to its horizons. That illusion, too, is the product of the eye-ear relationship.

For many years, doctors have used this relationship when examining small deaf-mute children. By rotating the child rapidly in a chair, they could induce nystagmus and giddiness provided the inner ear was intact. If nystagmus could not be induced, the probability was high that the ear labyrinth structures had been destroyed by injury or disease.

During the ENG examinations, Warren, while sitting on a table with the electrodes in place, was instructed to lie back with his head hanging over the table edge, and in "Hallpike maneuver" to move his head right, left, and up and down. A resulting benign vertigo would have indicated a normal condition. Warren's response was abnormal, but the source of the influence disturbing his nervous system continued to elude detection.

The boy's previous sight and hearing tests had been largely screening examinations that might have indicated the need for further, sophisticated probing. His hearing, already known to be normally acute, was now found to be normal in range as determined by cycles per second (CPS) examination.

A tangent screen test showed that blind spots were normally sized and located. These spots are caused by the retina's optical insensitivity at the point where it joins with the optic nerve. Perimetry provided an assessment of the visual field. For this, Warren sat in front of the device, looking straight ahead, and told the technician when he could and could not see 3-millimeter size red and white objects as they moved about the visual field. Pseudoisochromatics, a test involving colors and their tints, indicated that the boy had red-green color blindness. At the close of the first day, the source of Warren M.'s hyperactive symptoms remained an enigma.

The second day was largely devoted to the time-consuming five-hour glucose tolerance test. Other chemical tests made for the third day evaluations. The essential clue was discovered — and was isolated — on the third day. A carbon monoxide assay revealed a blood saturation at the dangerous 20 per cent level:

carbon monoxide toxicity was at least one source of Warren's problems.

It is always necessary to complete the workup so that no other causes go undiscovered, but the hyperactive child's diagnosis is typically found when diagnostic efforts are directed to associated biochemical test data. The biochemical testing area is a wide one. The presence or absence of anemia must be ascertained. To make this determination, the necessary laboratory data include the levels of the oxygen-bearing, iron-containing protein in the child's red blood cells, the lack of which causes anemia. The packing of the red blood cells following a centrifuge procedure is investigated. The normal level of the white blood cells ranges from 5000 to 10,000 per cubic millimeter of blood. This is tested by counting the cells of a diluted sampling under the microscope. The peripheral white cell count frequently provides a clue to intercurrent infection or allergy.

Often the proper metabolism of carbohydrates in the digestive process is suspect, causing diabetes or other sugar sensitivities, and so a five-hour glucose tolerance test may be helpful.

Other associated biochemical data are the serum levels of calcium and phosphorus (serum is the remaining blood when the red blood cells have been removed). Calcium, potassium, and magnesium salts are needed for cell polarity electrical balance in the central nervous system's cell membranes.

Many organ systems may influence the brain by their presence or absence in the blood of their end products. At this stage the liver, kidney, adrenal, and thyroid are assessed for the elevation or the depletion of their various beneficial or toxic products in the bloodstream.

However, Warren's first day's examinations had not been a waste of time and effort. The later biochemical, neurological, and hematological data are very individualized, and literally thousands of tests are possible. The logical sequence of each patient's neuropsychiatric workup directs the later stages of the examination to the likeliest cause or causes. Without the guidance of the neuropsychiatric data assembled during Warren's first day, thousands of biochemical tests might have been tried before the right one was hit upon.

More important, carbon monoxide poisoning, Warren's problem, is a major source of oxygenation problems. Oxygenation difficulties are frequently the cause of the hyperactivity syndrome. The brain's number-one priority is oxygen. Without oxygen, the brain cells cannot be nourished, nor can their waste products be carried away. Carbon monoxide and oxygen both combine with blood hemoglobin, but of the two carbon monoxide is more than two hundred times as strongly attracted to the red carrier pigment, so it displaces oxygen in the bloodstream. Chronic carbon monoxide intoxication may produce anoxic (absence of oxygen) effects throughout the body and affect the peripheral nerves more than the brain's cortex.

Warren's parents were asked to recheck their new house for possible sources of carbon monoxide, such as a deficient air supply to the oil-burning furnace or a defect in its venting. Warren was not to ride in the "old, jerky" school bus. He was cautioned also against his ear-popping habit, as this forcing of air from the throat into the Eustachian tubes could infect the inner ear.

Repeat studies three weeks later showed that Warren's carbon monoxide level had dropped to an acceptable 3 per cent. His behavioral difficulties resolved and he was again able to progress in his classroom studies. After a half-year interval, his EEG showed a marked improvement, with only slight residual abnormalities. Warren's eye movements were normal and his toxic color blindness was resolved. His mother telephoned other parents, encouraging them to attend a school board meeting. The board voted to purchase one new school bus and to replace the exhaust systems of three old ones. A neighbor's daughter then also ceased to suffer severe headaches.

When a Psychiatrist Is Needed

DR. JERRY NEWTON, AUTHOR OF AN EDITORIAL in the *Journal of the American Medical Association*, has suggested that physicians become more involved with aiding schools in the diagnosis and management of children with minimal brain damage (or dysfunction), hyperactivity, learning disability, and behavioral problems. Because medical education has neglected such problems, Dr. Newton believes that physicians view the syndrome as alien to their expertise. He notes: "These children have a serious disorder with an incidence quoted as 3% to 10% and, usually, with a poor prognosis." Nevertheless, he states that many physicians have helped by improving the causal classification and diagnostic methods of learning disability, and further says:

> An added benefit of increased physician involvement is that it offers a balance to the many spurious medically related nostrums that are advocated for children with learning disability and often eagerly accepted by the educational system: food coloring, crawling exercises, eye training, megavitamins, and hormones . . . We must ask ourselves why some of these remedies (so reminiscent of snake oil) become so widely accepted. It is because the voice of the physician is not heard in the land of education . . .[1]

Certainly most doctors engaged in general medical practice have little or no specialized training relating to the hyperactivity syndrome. There is, however, a group of physicians in the United States whose specialized training has been in that branch of the healing art to which medical schools expressly assign such problems as hyperactivity, minimal brain dysfunction, learning disability, and behavioral problems for study, diagnosis, and treatment. These men and women are, of course, psychiatrists.

By and large, how well qualified are psychiatrists to undertake the diagnosis and treatment of hyperactive children? Perhaps only a psychiatrist should answer this question. In Ellicott City, Maryland, Dr. Nelson Hendler told the 1976 Taylor Manor Psychiatric Symposium that psychiatrists "have lost the respect" of their fellow M.D.'s and the public and are not viewed as physicians by either group.

Dr. Hendler, of Johns Hopkins Hospital, Baltimore, charged at the same symposium that psychiatrists sometimes give treatments to a patient without having produced a diagnosis and without understanding the etiology of the symptoms. He believed that psychiatry has been hurt by its use of such new therapies as meditation, biofeedback, and acupuncture, as well as by its misuse of valuable modes of treatment.

Dr. Hendler further criticized psychiatrists for their abuse of medical responsibility in supervising community mental health centers. He said that in some cases psychiatrists have relied on the judgment of nurses, social workers, or mental health counselors without examining the patient themselves or without seeing a patient after the initial evaluation.

Hendler urged that psychiatrists become exceptional diagnosticians, capable of choosing a proper mode of treatment and serving as a consultant to other physicians. He said that in the role of consultant, the psychiatrist should offer information on psychotropic medication and warn of the psychotropic side effects of other drugs.

"Above all," Dr. Hendler said, the psychiatrist "should maintain a professional stature comparable with all of medicine. Only then will psychiatrists be considered physicians and put to good use the M.D. degree so essential to proper psychiatric care."[2]

Opinions very similar to those of Dr. Hendler were expressed by Dr. Myron G. Sandifer at the annual meeting of the American Psychiatric Association in Miami in 1976. Dr. Sandifer, professor of psychiatry and family practice at the University of Kentucky School of Medicine, Lexington, said that the psychiatrist should be able to perform certain general medical functions as well as to function in his specialty. At the head of the list of general medical functions Dr. Sandifer placed diagnostic evaluation.[3]

Quite obviously, the ranks of psychiatry contain diverse elements. There are wide differences in the theory, diagnosis, and the treatment of psychosis and psychoneurosis. Also, within the fellowship of psychiatry a new breed of practitioners and teachers is willing to recognize challenges, admit mistakes of the past, and will especially seek to repair the damage done by psychiatry's near-divorce from general medicine.

This new attitude is highly desirable in the treatment of the hyperactivity syndrome in childhood, for in so many cases the cause that must be diagnosed and treated is a physiological one and should be identified through adequate, modern neurological investigation rather than by probings of the patient's unconscious self.

Neurological and neuropsychiatric diagnosis is desirable also because it is open to the evidence gathered by objective tests and measurements. It is guided to its findings by what is discovered in the patient rather than by theoretical considerations in the diagnostician's mind. In the diagnosis of hyperactivity, SEG (which uses sonar waves to show any shift of the brain off its midline), EEG (to diagnose the brain's electrical activity), the brain scan, ophthalmodynamometry (a technique of measuring the adequacy of the blood circulation through the head), metachromic and opticokinetic findings (tests for colorblindness and for the brain-eye relationship), and biochemical investigative results count more than speculative conceptions.

Parents and teachers who may need to seek or to recommend psychotherapeutic help for a hyperactive child should be fully aware that the profession of psychiatry contains a number of splinter groups. I use the word "splinter" to describe the differing, exclusive modes of therapy that operate in a common sector. Thus, the sector of adult group psychotherapy includes transactional analysis, psychoanalytic, psychodrama, Gestalt, encounter, experiential-existential, and behavior group therapies. Each of these in its own way proposes to straighten out an individual's behavioral and emotional disorders.

All psychiatrists are not the same in the sense that brain surgeons, cardiologists, and urologists are alike; that is, alike in the admittedly wide sense that they specialize in definite areas of practice and employ recognized, if not standardized, modalities of treatment.

In an editorial written in early 1976, I touched upon the either-or attitude toward patients held by health care professionals and how this attitude tends to make "splitters" rather than "lumpers" in diagnosis.[4] (The effect of splitting is always to focus the diagnosis on one single finding. The effect of lumping is to gather *all* pertinent findings into a composite picture of what it is that causes the patient's condition.) Specifically, I cited the psychotherapist who may assume that differential diagnosis has taken place before the patient was referred for psychotherapy, and so supposes that the patient's possible physical problems have already been ruled out. (This is not necessarily true. The physician who made the referral may have acted on a hidden belief that "coping" problems invariably have psychogenic origins.)

Splitting occurs on a factional, or splinter, basis also. If our imaginary patient were an adult suffering much emotional distress, he or she might visit a half-dozen group psychotherapies and in each find a treatment unlike that in any of the others. Were the same patient to visit a half-dozen psychiatrists, he or she might conceivably be diagnosed in as many different ways because of the varying degrees of attention placed upon the "psyche" and the "soma" in psychosomatic diagnoses. A practitioner's adherence to the tenets of a splinter-group belief can narrow his or her field of vision in making a diagnosis. The same adherence is seen in the true believer's faith that some people bestow on fad drugs, herbs, and especially on diets.

Parents and teachers should consider the following points when they need to seek or recommend psychiatric assistance for a hyperactive child:

Will there be an accurate diagnosis preliminary to treatment? Any doctor, including a psychiatrist, who is lacking in enthusiasm for a broadly based, differential diagnosis — physiological, neurological, and psychiatric — will be unlikely to pursue thoroughly the numerous and diverse underlying causes of the hyperactivity syndrome.

Will there be a search for more than one underlying cause? A cause that is overlooked and goes untreated will continue to contribute to the child's problem, thereby preventing a cure.

Should the therapy be unproductive, will there be a search for an unidentified, ongoing cause that is somehow interfering with the treatment itself? If therapy is unproductive because a contributory cause has escaped being detected, it is important that the unidentified cause be identified for therapy to be successful. And it is certainly better to question the treatment than to write off the child as untreatable.

21

The Human Side of Hyperactivity

CLIFFORD V., A CASE HISTORY

Clifford V., a five-and-a-half-year-old allegedly retarded boy, was brought to the office by a juvenile protection agency social worker accompanied by the patient's foster mother. The social worker stated that the child was conceived during an estrangement when his natural mother and legal father were temporarily separated. The mother, living in Los Angeles at the time, had visited an agency there to discuss letting the child out for adoption, but she finally decided to keep her baby.

The infant was neglected, being totally rejected by the legal father. For the first twenty months of his life, Clifford was mostly confined to a crib in a back bedroom, infrequently changed, but left with a bottle. When given solid food, he was put on the floor with a dish and ate like an animal.

During a summer vacation period, the baby was left with another couple who were childless and who offered to adopt Clifford. After a few months in his new home, the child changed from being "dumb and lethargic" to a seemingly happy, active toddler. The adoptive parents were pleased with him, believed that he was unusually bright and that he was catching up rapidly. They felt that their experience was like seeing an old battered plaything turn into a bright new toy.

After the adoptive mother gave birth to a son, the couple

realized that their feelings about Clifford had changed. He was now someone else's kid that they were baby-sitting. He irritated the woman with his fussing, whining, fretful ways; he also was disobedient and seemed unable to learn anything. Just before his fifth birthday, Clifford was placed in foster care.

Up to this point, Clifford's behavioral development had been slow. Right-handed, he was poorly coordinated and couldn't ride a tricycle because he would push with both feet at the same time. With a pencil or crayon and paper he could do nothing but scribble. Though toilet-trained at age two-and-a-half, he was still soiling and unable to wipe himself after a bowel movement. Despite bladder training at age four, he was wetting himself and was severely spanked for it by his adoptive parents.

At two years he could say "mama" and "bye-bye" and at two-and-a-half years he could name a few objects. His adoptive parents reported that he talked gibberish. The social worker found him hard to understand and believed that in all situations he tended not to talk. His play behavior was reported as similarly retarded because of his short attention span and a tendency to scatter instead of play with toys.

At age five, he did not know any colors, could sometimes count to five, did not know any ABCs, and remained interested in TV for only about five minutes.

The adoptive parents stated that he loved to be babied, carried, and loved. They considered this "phony" on his part, and it turned them off. They found him to be a poor sleeper and a greedy eater who, if allowed to, would gorge until he vomited.

The foster mother's impressions were that in general Clifford functioned on the level of a three-year-old neighborhood child. He drank water excessively and always wanted to eat. She thought at first that he related better to her husband than to her. She felt that he was very curious about her behavior and her whereabouts, had very good manners, and knew how to brush his teeth. He still soiled his pants.

The foster mother found him very affectionate. Yet he didn't seem to remember verbal directions. She believed he enjoyed being in a Sunday school class with two- and three-year-olds.

The social worker said that she found Clifford an extremely appealing, lovable child. When she visited the adoptive home, he related at once to her and immediately sat on her lap. She thought he enjoyed going to visit the foster home, but he stayed close to her. After the first visit to the foster home, he knew the way and told her she should have turned at a certain corner when she took a different route. He liked individual attention, and several times when they were sitting quietly together he had said, "I love you." He frequently smiled at her as if expecting a smile of approval in return.

Shortly after moving to the foster home, Clifford fell and cut his head, requiring stitches. On this occasion he cried without making a sound. When the stitches came out, he did not say a word except to ask for a Band-Aid.

While the foster parents were away for a month, Clifford was placed in a vacation foster home. Here the temporary foster mother, who had had experience with difficult children, told the social worker that she did not believe Clifford was retarded, but he seemed to be tense about gaining approval.

In the fall, when Clifford started school, he was reported as spitting on girls, being "up and down" in class, still not knowing colors, and unable to get along with other children of his age, so that the teacher finally sent him home — put him on one hour in school a day. By October the teacher felt that Clifford could do more when he wanted to and would "come across if you let him know you won't accept infantile behavior." In tests, he was performing at about the three-and a-third-year-old level. His attention span was better in small groups. When excited, he "went wild," hitting others on the head.

Clifford's medical history included inoculations: diphtheria times three, polio times three, measles, mumps, and rubella. No smallpox. He had been tested for tuberculosis on three occasions. He had had hernia repair in infancy, had been evaluated for possible hypothyroidism, and had had an EEG that was considered mildly abnormal. He had had severe bronchitis, episodes of high fever, and a bone x ray. Aside from past ear infections, a high frequency of bowel movements, transient periods of wetting himself, and questionable itching, the review of systems was noncontributory. Other than the questionable descent of testes bilaterally, the general physical examination was likewise noncontributory.

As the examination proceeded, significant findings appeared in emotional reactions (laughs appropriately, does weep, although silently), manners of relating (an affectionate boy who has had difficulty relating to other children in the past), and character of play (prefers to play with dolls, although he had recently mastered a tricycle).

Associated biochemical data, however, revealed an elevated sed rate of 34. In this very simple procedure, a blood sample is placed in a test tube for an hour and the rate at which red blood cells fall indicates the loss of cell coating. An elevated rate thus points to some disease or infectious condition in the patient. Clifford had a magnesium count of 1.6, below the normal range of 1.8–2.5. A deficiency of magnesium may cause symptoms of anxiety, apprehension, agitation, and confusion and in severe cases can appear as psychiatric disorders.

The impressions were:

1. Normal neurological evaluation, as the EEG findings were normal for Clifford's age.
2. Mental retardation would be doubtful in view of number 1.
3. Hypomagnesmia would probably reflect a poor intake of magnesium because of inadequate nutrition, and a loss of magnesium because of the boy's overly active bowel condition.
4. Contributing pathological, emotional, and developmental abnormalities show the baneful effects of child neglect and abuse, whether involving physical or mental cruelty. Babies need to be picked up, cuddled, talked to, sung to, played with. People must reach out to children or children will never learn how to reach out to people.

I recommended the following:

1. Maintain a well-balanced nutritional status.
2. Involve Clifford with kindergarten activities in which he can succeed at his present state of development and through which he will be able to mingle with other children on an equal basis.

3. Reevaluate the magnesium and sed rates in three to six months.
4. I would like to write a prescription for Clifford, calling for large daily doses of caring attention from understanding foster parents supplemented by the instruction of a patient and perceptive teacher.

NORMAN A., A CASE HISTORY

Norman A. was brought in when he was nine years and nine months old by his mother for a neurological evaluation directed to his difficulties — his headaches, his stomachaches, and the ringing in his ears. These ills were coupled with more problems in school and at home.

Norman's present symptoms were first described in a letter from Mrs. A., who lived in a western state where, she wrote, she could not find a doctor who would give her son the complete examination necessary to evaluate his condition properly. She said that she had a friend in Southern California with whom she could stay for whatever time was needed to make a diagnosis.

A second letter was more insistent: "There is something very wrong with Norman physically. He complains all the time of headaches, he is very nervous, and also constantly has horrible sores in his mouth, usually accompanied with a rash over his body (which primarily occurs in the areas of his joints), and he has a foul odor on his breath that does not seem to be simply bad breath, but rather from his stomach." She added that she had taken the boy to a pediatrician, who simply prescribed Ritalin, "which does nothing but make him a 'zombie' for a couple of hours at a time, mostly when he is in school, because I refuse to give it to him at home. Norman is also being seen by a psychiatrist once a week. Frankly, to my knowledge this is not the solution, either." This second letter was signed Mrs. K.U., with the explanation that her son's father, a defense contractor, had died while in Alaska. The friend with whom she planned to stay was a former Alaskan acquaintance.

During the ensuing three-day examination, Norman's headaches were described as having started approximately three years before, after a concussion he suffered at age six. The ringing in the ears was primarily in the right ear, usually noticed in the afternoon, not associated with deafness or a sensation of fullness, but occasionally accompanied by nausea. There was no manifest vomiting, motion sickness, or ear infection. The stomachaches were described as ongoing, with tendencies to constipation and to diarrhea, again with no associated nausea or vomiting.

There was no known diabetes in the family. The boy's tantrums occurred primarily in the morning and were mitigated with eating.

Norman typically went to bed between nine o'clock and ninethirty. He had difficulty falling asleep and slept lightly and restlessly, with frequent night terrors. There was no night soiling. He was unrefreshed in the morning, ate only toast or a doughnut with milk and coffee at breakfast, was driven to school, and carried a sandwich for lunch. At dinner, between six and seven o'clock, he showed a good appetite.

Norman's developmental history began with a normal ninemonth gestation. As a baby he was bottle-fed, and was described as a poor sucker with frequent vomiting. He sat between eight and nine months, walked at eighteen months, talked at one year, and was toilet-trained at two years. He was right-handed. He attended preschool and was described as hitting and scratching his peers. His kindergarten experience was similar. In the third grade, he was placed in a special educational program. He practiced pica.

Norman's inoculation history was a typical inclusive one. He had frequent sore throats, and he had had high temperatures accompanied by feverish convulsions. The medical history recorded no childhood diseases, but he had spent a week in the hospital at age one and a half for vomiting and diarrhea, and had had his tonsils and adenoids removed at age six.

Norman's father died at age thirty-five in an aircraft crash. He had been typically in good health, as were the boy's mother and his seventeen-year-old half sister.

Norman now lived in a suburban townhouse with electric

baseboard heating; he had no pets and engaged in no hobbies. The boy had his own room, but there was a history of his sleeping frequently in his mother's room.

His mother explained that Norman feared many strange things, such as empty rooms and balloons, and when he heard an airplane overhead he would run, scream, and try to hide. In heavy automobile traffic, he had shown the same frightened response. On one occasion, after Norman was asleep for the night, he awoke screaming, exhibited violent behavior accompanied by the vomiting of yellowish fluid, after which he ran screaming incoherently around the house. After calming down somewhat, he complained of a headache across the front of his head and was very nervous and hyperactive. Another day, his mother described her pregnancy as a period of great emotional stress between herself and her husband, stating that when six months pregnant she had received a kick in her stomach during a quarrel with Norman's father.

Norman's general physical examination was essentially noncontributory. The neurological examination revealed a more than normal blood supply of the optic disks in both eyes, with an eye muscle weakness also. Associated biochemical data revealed a mildly abnormal response to the five-hour glucose tolerance test as well as elevated presence of calcium and phosphorus, low carbon dioxide, and borderline sodium presence.

The impressions in this diagnostic effort were numerous, incorporating many findings of abnormalities of varying, and difficult to assess, severity:

1. Mild to moderate cortical lability, disclosed by EEG recordings.
2. Labyrinthine instability, disclosed by electronystagmograph eye nerve–inner ear relationship.
3. Hyperventilation, abnormal excessive breathing with buzzing in the ears, sometimes with fainting, which in Norman's case was associated with anxiety, affecting impressions 1 and 2.
4. Mild but possible contributing carbohydrate abnormality.
5. Possible hypercalcemia must be ruled out.
6. Pathological child-parent relationship as secondary to unresolved Oedipal phenomenon in a fatherless family situation.

I recommended the following:

1. Stabilize the cortical-labyrinthine instability with diphenylhydantoin, 50 mg twice a day.
2. Correct diet, avoiding excessive carbohydrates.
3. Avoid Norman's sleeping in his mother's bedroom by a situational adjustment.
4. Reevaluate the abnormal biochemical parameters in four weeks.

The Southern California Neuropsychiatric Institute files contain a note received some months following: "Thank you for your help. My son, Norman, is doing fine. I shall be grateful to Dr. Walker for the rest of my life. Please thank him for me." This, as I view it, is not a personal tribute but an acknowledgment of the superiority of differential neuropsychiatric diagnosis over indiscriminate stimulant drug pill popping.

HENRY Y., A CASE HISTORY

Henry Y. was brought in by his mother for a neurological evaluation in relation to the child's ongoing difficulties with hyperactive behavior, flawed learning achievement, and urinary distress. The boy, seven years and seven months old, had a long-standing and continuing habit of nightly bedwetting, which had not been overcome by a meatal dilation of the urinary passage, or by his taking Ritalin for a year.

Mrs. Y. stated that Henry first demonstrated uncontrolled behavior when he was in kindergarten, showing random uneasiness and a poor attention span. She believed that, though he had no great difficulty getting along with other children his age, he preferred being alone.

The boy was described as going reluctantly and protestingly to bed, typically around seven-thirty, and sleeping deeply until awakening at seven, appearing refreshed. His eating habits reflected no food faddism. His daytime behavior did not suggest fatigue or a breakdown in his coordination. (This was asserted early in the interview. Later, during the review of systems, he was described as being somewhat uncoordinated.)

Henry was not able to sit quietly during the review of information. His early development was somewhat precocious. He was described as possessing extraordinary energy from an early age and, indeed, was reputed to have raised his head at birth. He sat at seven months, stood at ten months, and walked at a year. For the first three months of life he was breast-fed and had no difficulty sucking. The mother recalled his having questionable colic and said that he was not a cuddly baby.

Henry had the usual inoculations. He ran temperatures of 105 degrees without feverish convulsions. His medical history was without measles, chicken pox, mumps, rheumatic fever, or scarlet fever. He had never been hospitalized for any medical or surgical cause. There was no known history of heart disease, kidney disease, tuberculosis, liver disease, bone or joint disease, sugar in his urine, high blood pressure, or any allergy recognized as such.

His parents were in generally good health; the mother, however, had ongoing endometriosis, an inflammation of the uterine mucous membrane. One of Henry's sisters had ear infections, and a younger brother had hernias and a bed-wetting problem. His other siblings were in good health. Both grandfathers had died of heart diease, both grandmothers of cancer; a great-aunt had tuberculosis and an uncle had high blood pressure.

In addition to the foregoing family history, details subsequently recalled contained references to allergies affecting Henry's father, his siblings, and a maternal uncle, as well as paternal cousins with asthma. Henry himself, by skin test indications, had sensitivities to rye grass, brome grass, lamb's quarters, and oak, walnut, and elm trees. Among foods tested, he had significant reactions to nuts, especially walnut, pecan and Brazil nuts. He also reacted to eating coconut and among other foods causing milder reactions were chocolate, melons, rye, wheat, squash, tomatoes, pears, shrimp, cow's milk, and raw beef.

The review of systems in Henry's case was apparently noncontributory, aside from complaints of chest pains and his problem with enuresis.

The general physical examination was not noteworthy except for a hair whorl on the right. This detail was associated with a finding of possible mixed dominance in the right-handed, right-eyed, but left-footed child who had a persistent problem with reversals such as "d" for "b" and other reading difficulty. The associated neurophysiologic data revealed a mildly abnormal EEG (because of dysrhythmic quality and transient episodes of slowing) and a mildly abnormal ENG.

The associated biochemical data showed an abnormal response in the five-hour glucose tolerance study and disclosed an elevated eosinophilia, a numerically minor white blood cell group whose numbers increase in the presence of allergies and parasitic infections.

The impressions were:

1. Mild to moderate cortical lability, as revealed by an EEG, showing brain surface electrical . activity.
2. Mild to moderate labyrinthine instability, as demonstrated by ENG finding of eye–inner ear problems.
3. Carbohydrate abnormality. Mild to moderate, affecting #1 and #2.
4. Possible hereditary allergic predisposition, affecting impressions 1 and 2.

I recommended the following:

1. Challenge carbohydrate abnormality with removal of carbohydrates from Henry's diet.
2. Reevaluate eosinophilia (white blood cell presence) when normal regimen has been achieved.

Henry's difficulties were *not* resolved through this treatment. This is not to say that these problems did not exist. They *did*, and they *were* resolved, but they were not all of the underlying, determining causes of Henry's hyperactivity and learning disability problem.

It might, of course, be that his being treated with Ritalin at the time of his diagnosis could in some degree have blurred the findings.

Again, it may simply be that the examination was made at the three-quarter mark of the twentieth century. The year 1984, to say nothing of the year 2000, is some while distant. In laboratories today, men and women are searching out the secrets of the human body's cells and cellular processes and the mysteries of the membranes. It is quite possible that Henry Y. is the victim of some now-suspected dysfunction of a membrane's permeability, which bars or deflects the transmitting of an autonomic nervous system impulse. In the management of the hyperactivity syndrome, as everywhere in medicine, progress is yet to be made, thresholds are still to be crossed.

Arne C., a Case History

Arne C. was brought in by his mother following a preliminary interview with Mr. C., an import company executive. The boy's mother appeared to be a reliable source of information. She stated that Arne, now nineteen years old, was born in Hawaii, where the family had been living, and that the baby's behavior first seemed unusual while nursing, when he would be easily startled. By approximately six months, he was fussy without definite colic. Mrs. C. could recall no infections, high temperatures, or head traumas during this period.

At around age three, Arne progressively demonstrated an interest in wrapping himself in a blanket and rocking. It was also at this age that he developed an apparent sleeping disorder, awakening during the night to sing and laugh to himself for a while before going back to sleep.

The child's first spoken words were precocious, occurring at six months. However, his meaning and thought took on a strict mimicry and repetition and avoided the use of nouns. The expression "All dark outside, honey" was used to express a wish to look out the window, and "Don't you want some ketchup, honey?" was used to ask for something to eat.

Progressively, Arne showed a rhythmic and rigid behavioral pattern. There were violent outbursts when he was not allowed to follow his routine, even when slight changes in the expected order occurred. He displayed a marked fondness for music and had good rhythm.

His hunger was persistent. He had a urinary infection at age four without complaints of soreness. Arne had no history of either dizziness or of ringing in his ears, but he did get carsick, even without looking out the window.

During his early developmental years, Arne typically went to bed at approximately seven o'clock, falling asleep with ease, sleeping deeply, and awakening during the small hours. It was at this time that he rocked, sang, and laughed to himself without demanding attention from others. He would awaken again at approximately five o'clock, feeling refreshed. He ate a hearty breakfast, usually of cereal, eggs, milk, and fruit. Then he would start his ritualistic activities. These included bobbing in a chair, swaying, wrapping himself up, rocking, and assembling and disassembling the vacuum cleaner. Attempts to interrupt this pattern resulted in screaming. There was a change in the child's appearance and alertness accompanied by a "glassy" look during his episodes of automatic behavior. The boy ate lunch readily, again showing a good appetite. He took an hour-and-a-half nap during the afternoon. Upon his waking, the repetitive behavior resumed, with screaming and crying if things were not in the proper order or if he was interrupted. At dinner Arne showed a good appetite without food preferences.

Arne's developmental history began with a normal nine-month gestation, during which time his mother gained 16 pounds. She was under the care of a doctor. She had no high blood pressure, protein in her urine, or seizures. Labor was spontaneous and lasted three hours. Birth was without anesthesia, the mother being alert at the time of delivery. The infant was presented head first and breathed spontaneously. His birth weight was 5 pounds, 13 ounces.

Throughout his early developmental history, Arne had no record of unusual weight loss or gain. There was no postprandial sweating, urinary tract infection before age four, boils, styes, or excessive thirst. After his precocious first words at six months, he regressed and did not start meaningful speech until age eight. At eight years, also, he was toilet-trained.

Arne received the usual inoculations. Tine was negative as to tuberculosis. The boy had chicken pox, but not measles, mumps, rheumatic fever, or scarlet fever; he had not been hospitalized and had not had high temperatures with feverish convulsions. At approximately age seven, he suffered a chronic skin condition, ultimately diagnosed as persistent flea bites, which did not affect any other member of the family.

Arne had episodes of asthma between ages six and ten. He had no medical history of heart, liver, kidney, bone, or joint disease nor any history of high blood pressure, seizures, tuberculosis, diabetes, or loss of consciousness. (That a patient has no medical history of an ailment does not mean that he or she has never had the illness or condition, only that its presence has never been observed and diagnosed so that it could be recorded.)

In the course of the attempted management of his behavioral problem by psychotherapeutic modes, Arne received only routine medical attention for his physical and physiological difficulties. An amphetamine drug was given and was believed to have helped modify his childhood tantrums. Later, thyroid therapy was given. When I first examined him, the youth was on a megavitamin schedule made up of B, C, and E vitamins.

Turning to his family medical history, both parents had reached middle age in good health, but Arne's fifteen-year-old brother had a terminal blood disease. Twin sisters, age eleven, were in good health. A grandmother had had cancer, two grandfathers were diabetic, and there were great-aunts and great-uncles having or having had arthritis, gout, and thyroid problems.

Ever since, at around age eight, Arne developed some meaningful speech, he had been gradually placed in individual tutoring situations. At the time of this diagnosis he was functioning at the 6½-grade level. He had been reading for pleasure since about age twelve. More recently he had shown an interest in athletics. He performed his household chores regularly and dependably.

My general physical examination revealed an abnormality of excessive blood supply to the eye disk on the left, a poor reaction to direct light, and an eye muscle weakness. Some of his reflexes were deficient or doubtful. His neurological examination showed some failures to develop normally in these areas.

Associated neurophysiological data revealed an abnormal EEG, an abnormal ENG, and defects of vision as shown in an abnormal tangent screen. Associated biochemical data revealed problems of liver functioning and an abnormal response to the five-hour glucose tolerance test in the first hour.

The impressions were:

1. Chronic brain syndrome, shown by history of behavior and learning disability and by EEG.
2. Inner-ear instability, as disclosed in history, examination, and ENG.
3. Possible contributing carbohydrate abnormality disclosed by glucose tolerance test.
4. Possible contributing Brill's disease (a form of typhus) in the light of fleabite history.

I recommended the following:

1. Stabilize the carbohydrate problem by correcting Arne's diet. Healthy eating patterns are already established.
2. Consider stabilization of the inner-ear labyrinth with antihistamine as needed.
3. Consider further investigation of the carbohydrate problem with studies of amino acid (protein) sensitivity or milk-sugar sensitivity.

The outcome was gratifying. Arne had been largely unresponsive to psychotherapeutic ministration so long as his pressing physiological deficiencies and disorders were going undetected and untreated. Following neuropsychiatric diagnosis and appropriate medical attention, he has stabilized to a level that permits him to attend school and function successfully in the remedial classroom environment. The prognosis now is that he will achieve self-sufficiency eventually.

22

Parents' Resources and the Future

HYPERACTIVITY AS A MAJOR PERIL to the nation's children first surfaced in the public schools, and in individual cases is still at least half of the time first identified in the schoolroom. The syndrome creates educational problems. It is not itself an educational problem, and there is not much that public schools can be expected to do for hyperactive children that is not already being done. Local boards of education are almost everywhere hard pressed to cope with current building costs, salary demands, threatened strikes by teachers and noncertificated employees, and the expenses of racial desegregation programs.

Moreover, even if no financial problems were involved, school boards, superintendents, school psychologists, teaching specialists, and classroom teachers, while they may not like drugging children, seem to be unaware of any alternative. They appear reluctant to consider the possibility that an alternative exists. In these circumstances, it is not surprising that many parents have turned to do-it-yourself diagnosis in treating their youngsters' behavioral and learning difficulties. It is worth noting here that even doctors themselves do not diagnose and treat members of their own family. The risks of their professional judgment being warped by personal involvement are too serious to be chanced.

Realistically, what parents can do for a hyperactive child depends upon their sagacity — and it may be their stick-to-it-iveness also — in seeking professional assistance. Certainly only physicians with special training and experience whose skills and insights are supplemented by sophisticated technical resources should be chosen to resolve the subtle problems of a hyperactive child. Your first goal as a parent is to find a physician in whom you can be fully confident.

If you leave your hyperactive child in the hands of the family doctor, his or her problems will be treated in the light of that physician's possibly limited expertise. The wiser course may be to ask the general practitioner to recommend a specialist for you to consult. Make it clear to the family doctor, and to whatever specialist he or she may refer you, that you want a search made for a physiological cause underlying your youngster's behavioral symptoms — a cause that could be organic, metabolic, or toxic.

The responsibility for choosing an appropriate treatment for your child rests with you. Parents who are not adequately informed risk spending a good deal of money and time just to find out that their child is still in the Ritalin rut after mediocre diagnosis and treatment. Being aware of the perils of do-it-yourself diagnosis is not enough. Being aware of the shortcomings of office call, stethoscope, and reflex-hammer is not enough. Nor is it sufficient to realize that books — this one included — or health-oriented magazines cannot tell you how to diagnose and treat your child. Groups composed of well-intentioned parents whose children have been helped by one or another treatment cannot advise you unbiasedly on how to treat your child's individual problem.

What is required of you?

It is necessary to keep in mind that your child's hyperactive behavior is not in itself the problem, but is only a *symptom* arising from a source or several sources that must be accurately diagnosed and properly treated. The child's behavior can be likened to an adult's pacing the floor, which is a mild form of grown-up hyperactivity that may stem from a toothache, a financial crisis, or the agony of waiting for a jury to bring in its verdict. A tranquilizer may temporarily soothe the adult's agitation, but it won't mend the decayed tooth, avert bankruptcy, or influence the jury. Similarly, merely treating a child's hyperactivity *symptom* does nothing to heal the underlying problem or problems, which possibly include an ongoing and worsening disorder.

Parents should be prepared for stumbling blocks along the way to obtaining comprehensive diagnosis and appropriate treatment. Most members of the medical profession still believe, practice, and in some prominent instances teach, as though treatment of the hyperactivity syndrome were limited to its being "managed" by alleviative measures that include stimulant drugs or, rarely, tranquilizers. Your family doctor will probably refer you to one of these veteran practitioners. It isn't a question of the physician's age, however. Even many young doctors believe in drug therapy, having become only barely acquainted with the existence of hyperactivity during their training.

If you specify that what you have in mind is an orthodox pediatrician who will base your child's treatment on a comprehensive, differential examination and specific diagnosis, you just might be referred to an excellent child specialist. Your child might well benefit on the other hand from the services of a thoroughly capable and conscientious neurologist, a specialist in dealing with the nervous system and its disorders. Whatever specialist you consult, be aware that many doctors do not make all the necessary tests or do them sloppily. Even among adult patients, I keep finding serious disorders that have not been completely or adequately evaluated by their previous physicians.

To avoid this, be present throughout the neurological examination, ask questions, and require adequate responses to them. Answering questions is part of every physician's duties, and here particularly, the extent to which the father or the mother is an informed parent is important to the child's welfare. The book you now hold in your hands will guide you along the course of an adequate, differential diagnostic examination (see chapter 19).

Some parents are severely handicapped by living in communities distant from neurologists and pediatricians; many localities do not have a general practitioner. In these circumstances, the best course may be to turn to the medical school of your state university. You should direct queries to the medical school's departments of neurology, psychiatry, and pediatrics. You will want your child to be seen by resident doctors, interns, and medical students as a patient in the school's clinic.

Research findings from some medical schools have figured significantly in changing the attitudes of doctors and educators toward stimulant drugs from one of uncritical acceptance to that of an increasing degree of restraint. They haven't gone far enough or fast enough, but the move has recently been in the right direction. Though your state's university may not have participated in such projects, the medical school faculty are likely to be well aware of the latest developments in the field. Certainly it is reasonable to expect that as more hyperactive children are seen by today's medical students, interns, and residents — particularly as more of these children are examined in the departments of neurology — the better diagnosis and treatment will be in the years ahead. We may see fewer and fewer top neurologists and pediatricians clinging to the belief that medical examinations, EEGs, and detection of sensory defects are irrelevant in evaluating hyperactivity.

It would however be utterly unrealistic to suppose that the problems of millions of children are going to be solved by referrals from family doctors and admissions to university medical school clinics. At present, the children whose needs can be met are the youngsters who have dedicated, persistent, persuasive parents — parents who are thoroughly convinced of the need for differential diagnosis as a basis for treatment and will follow through in pursuing this for their child.

The problem is not to persuade people to use existing neurological and neuropsychiatric facilities. The problem is to persuade the public and public officials that there must be more of these facilities, and that the great majority of hyperactive youngsters (who are not being seen by physicians or receiving treatment of any kind) must make use of them for diagnosis and treatment. As early as 1972, Gerald Solomons proposed that regional centers should be established to which hyperactive children could go for diagnosis. In the same year, Dr. Virginia Apgar stated that the diagnosis of these children would ideally take place in special diagnostic centers or in the medical departments of principal universities. (Yet even in some of these universities the most active advocates of treating children with stimulant drugs can be found.)

A nationwide system of regional diagnostic centers could indeed contribute to a brighter future for hyperactive youngsters, but only if the service provided is truly *diagnostic* in the widest sense; it must provide a completely comprehensive, meticulous neuropsychiatric examination and evaluation.

That will not happen if the project is entrusted to the people who gave us methylphenidate and other alleviative treatments that, in the light of recent critical studies, have failed to affect significantly the dismal long-term outcomes for the hyperactive child.

Neither is it likely that medical schools will set up diagnostic centers, independent and apart from their departments of psychiatry. Still less is it likely that any branch of government can create a system of such centers without being subjected to pressures from the drug industry, which has a financial stake in the management of hyperactivity, and by the trade journals, which have a stake in the advertising of pharmaceutical products, and by those individuals who, for profit's sake or on principle, fear and oppose socialized medicine.

Neverthless, the future is not altogether gloomy. Parents can be a power to be reckoned with. By a 1975 National Center for Educational Statistics report, there were in that year 3.5 million hyperactive children. Most of them were not being seen by doctors or receiving treatment of any kind. To date, the political influence that 7 million parents might exert on behalf of their children remains only potential. Little is heard from or about organized groups for the advancement of hyperactive children's interests and programs.

If you know of such a club, league, or study group, you would do well to join it. If there is no active organization in the area, you could get one started. Your child and other hyperactive children will benefit. Parent groups can improve the lives of hyperactive children by bringing the needs of their youngsters to the attention of boards of education, the town or city councils, and other governmental organizations. Active organizations of parents of hyperactive children will not lack for warm discussion of new and novel treatments. What parents can wisely do in these discussions is ask questions, become informed, and be skeptical of all cure-alls, whether they be Ritalin, a more recent drug, or a diet.

One subject parent groups should consider is "over-utilization," a term insurance companies apply when, in the company's opinion, a physician orders too many medical tests. Some unconscionable physicians order all possible tests and use none of the data. Some — not all — insurance companies may balk at paying the bills. As a parent, your concern is that nothing be overlooked when your child is diagnosed, that no opportunity to explore medical clues be passed by. Here your parent group may be valuable, for other parents may have had experience with various insurance companies and their policies in respect to "over-utilization."

Throughout the United States, patients who by reason of strokes or injuries or disease need an EEG, an ENG, or blood tests find that the necessary facilities are available — although expensive and not always located within the patient's immediate vicinity. A medical system that can provide services to individuals, young or old, who are afflicted by paralysis or have been injured, or who have one or another disease, can surely be able to provide the same services to hyperactive children — children who, if they are not helped, face the likelihood of alcohol or drug abuse, lifelong deprivation, depression, sometimes of eventual psychosis.

Neuropsychiatric diagnosis and the treatment sometimes required to remedy a subtle disorder can be expensive, yet it is cheaper by far than the human, social, and financial costs of uneducable children who will become adolescent delinquents and who in adult years will be likely to spend lifetimes as welfare charges since they will be unemployable due to lack of education and persistent ill-health.

There are portents of change. One is the class action suit filed by the Youth Center of San Francisco against the Taft, California, City School District. That this may be only the first of many such suits to be filed against school districts is strongly suggested by a paper, "Children's Rights: The Legal Aspects of Drugs and the Hyperactive Child," presented at an Operation Learning Conference in May of 1976 by Joseph Fleming.[1]

Mr. Fleming, a legal intern at the New York University Urban Law Clinic, stated that the Washington Square Legal Services Corporation, through the Urban Law Clinic, is engaged in a project to evaluate the legal ramifications of the use of drugs to control the behavior of schoolchildren. He pointed to the possibility of legal measures apparently far exceeding the scope of the Taft class action suit. He predicted that as long-run effects of psychoactive drugs begin to appear, "a lot of doctors, a lot of teachers, and, yes, a lot of parents may find themselves on the short end of a jury verdict." Fleming asserted that the ultimate protector and enforcer of the child's rights is not the parent but the state. He cited a case in which a mother sought to force her fifteen-year-old daughter to have an abortion. The court held that neither the mother nor the state could compel the minor child to submit, thus recognizing the right of a child to refuse intrusion into her body. With reference to psychoactive drugs, he asserted that the Washington Square Legal Services Corporation, as a child's guardian, could enforce the child's right not to have his or her body invaded by foreign substances whose long-range effects are not yet known. Other efforts in drug medication control promised by Mr. Fleming involved the fields of legislation, regulation, and negotiation.

It is not possible to assess the effects of court decisions that have not yet been rendered. Neither is it possible to predict the consequences of impending or threatened court actions in relation to the already onerous burden of malpractice insurance borne by the medical profession. Yet it does seem possible that the financial risks to a family physician of prescribing stimulant drugs will be far out of proportion to the income from this area of practice.

A much more significant deterrent will be the growing recognition by doctors that such medication does not meet the long-range needs of the young hyperactive patient. The deterrent will lie in the growing awareness of hyperactivity's serious implications. Parent groups could work to increase their awareness. In the words of Dr. Kenneth Swainan, chairman of the division of pediatric neurology at the University of Minnesota Medical School in Minneapolis, "The family practitioner doesn't pretend to be able to help the children with the complex problems that we treat." Certainly the future of the hyperactive child will brighten with the quickening recognition among family doctors that the syndrome presents complex difficulties that cannot be resolved by current modes of alleviative drug therapy. It follows that children with behavioral and learning disabilities should be referred for appropriate diagnosis before treatment is prescribed.

Indeed, the day may not be distant when those parents and teachers who are quite contented with drug-induced "good" behavior will find physicians declining to write prescriptions for those drugs.

Yet, at the present time, it is up to the intelligent and conscientious parent to insist upon an adequate diagnosis of the child. You have the right to choose a mode of diagnosis that is broad, precise, penetrating, and balanced in considering the multiple organic, infectious, neurological, endocrine-metabolic, genetic, and environmental factors. Any one of these, or several in combination, may be the underlying cause of your small son's or daughter's hyperactive symptoms.

BRAND AND GENERIC NAMES
FOR DRUGS CITED

NOTES

INDEX

Brand and Generic Names For Drugs Cited

Brand name	Generic name
Aventyl	protriptyline
Benadryl	diphenhydramine
Benzedrine	amphetamine sulfate
Dexedrine	dextroamphetamine
Dilantin	diphenylhydantoin
Eskalith	lithium carbonate
Ritalin	methylphenidate
Stelazine	trifluperazine
Thorazine	chlorpromazine
Tofranil	imipramine

Notes

Chapter 1.
Childhood's Life-Crippling Affliction   (pp. 3–14)

1. Paul H. Wender, M.D., "Peck's Bad Boys — A Growing Concern," *U.S. News and World Report*, May 27, 1974, pp. 72–75.
2. T. Berry Brazelton, M.D., "The Children Who Can't Sit Still," *Redbook*, August 1972, p. 72 et seq.
3. HEW–OCD Report, *JLD* 4: 61. (Office of Child Development Report on the Conference on the Use of Stimulant Drugs in the Treatment of Behaviorally Disturbed Young School Children, 1971. Reprinted in *Journal of Learning Disabilities* 4, no. 9 (November 1971): 59–66.)
4. Beverly J. Small, "The Hyperactive Child," *Today's Education*, January–February 1974, pp. 34–36.
5. Peter Schrag and Diane Divoky, *The Myth of the Hyperactive Child & Other Means of Child Control* (New York, Pantheon Books, 1975), p. 35.
6. Barbara K. Keough, "Hyperactivity and Learning Problems: Implications for Teachers," *Academic Therapy* 7 (fall 1971), pp. 47–50; *Education Digest*, December 1971, pp. 45–47.
7. Mark A. Stewart, M.D., in a 1975 address before the American Academy of Child Psychiatrists, California Medical Association.
8. Joseph N. Murray, "Drugs to Control Classroom Behavior," *Education Leadership* 31 (October 1973), pp. 21–25; *Education Digest*, January 1974, pp. 13–15.
9. Dorothea M. Ross and Sheila A. Ross, *Hyperactivity: Research-Theory-Action* (New York, John Wiley, 1976), p. 265.

10. J. Gordon Millichap, M.D., *The Hyperactive Child with Minimal Brain Dysfunction: Questions and Answers* (Chicago, Yearbook Medical Publishers, Inc., 1975), p. 35.
11. Dennis P. Cantwell, M.D., ed., et al., *The Hyperactive Child: Diagnosis, Management, Current Research* (New York, Spectrum Publications, Inc. 1976), pp. 51–63.
12. Wallace Mendelson, M.D., Noel Johnson, M.D., and Mark A. Stewart, M.D., "Hyperactive Children as Teenagers: A Follow-up Study," *Journal of Nervous and Mental Disease* 153, no. 4, pp. 273–279.
13. UPI, "Learning Ills, Crime Linked," San Diego *Evening Tribune*, p. D-1.

Chapter 2.
A History of Hyperactivity (pp. 15–26)

1. Charles Bradley, M.D., "The Behavior of Children Receiving Benzedrine," *American Journal of Psychiatry* 94 (November 1937): 577–585.
2. Ibid., p. 582.
3. Mark A. Stewart, M.D. and Sally Wendkos Olds, *Raising a Hyperactive Child* (New York, Harper & Row, 1973), p. 236.
4. *Scientific American*, July 1974, p. 39.
5. Charles Bradley, M.D., and Margaret Bowen, R.N., "Amphetamine (Benzedrine) Therapy of Children's Behavior Disorders," *American Journal of Orthopsychiatry*, January 1941, pp. 92–103.
6. Ibid., pp. 98–99.
7. J. Gordon Millichap, M.D., *The Hyperactive Child with Minimal Brain Dysfunction: Questions and Answers* (Chicago, Yearbook Medical Publishers, 1975), p. 100.
8. Harlan Vinnedge, "Drugs for Children." *New Republic*, March 13, 1971, pp. 13–15.
9. HEW–OCD Report, *JLD* 4, no. 9, pp 59–63.
10. Peter J. Ognibe, "Amphetamines and Barbiturates," *New Republic*, February 3, 1973, pp. 21–23.
11. Peter Schrag and Diane Divoky, *The Myth of the Hyperactive Child* (New York, Pantheon Books, 1975), p. 89.
12. Anita Johnson, "Greasing the Skids for Approval," *The Nation*, November 2, 1974, pp. 435–436.
13. "Even Millionaires Have Money Problems," *Forbes*, July 1, 1974, p. 22.

Chapter 3.
Who Becomes Hyperactive? *(pp. 27—32)*

1. J. Gordon Millichap, M.D., *The Hyperactive Child with Minimal Brain Dysfunction: Questions and Answers* (Chicago, Yearbook Medical Publishers, Inc., 1975), p. 8.
2. Ben F. Feingold, M.D., *Why Your Child Is Hyperactive* (New York, Random House, 1975), pp. 6–14.
3. Joseph N. Murray, "Drugs to Control Classroom Behavior," *Education Leadership* 31 (October 1973), pp. 21–25; *Education Digest*, January 1974, pp. 13–15.
4. Mark A. Stewart, M.D., and Sally Wendkos Olds, *Raising a Hyperactive Child* (New York, Harper and Row, 1973), p. 19.
5. Sydney Walker, III, M.D., *Psychiatric Signs and Symptoms Due to Medical Problems* (Springfield, Ill., Charles C. Thomas, 1967), pp. 205–209.

Chapter 5.
The Search for Underlying Causes *(pp. 43–52)*

1. Anita Miller, "A Woman Ought to Know," San Diego *Evening Tribune*, December 23, 1976, p. D-1.

Chapter 6.
Pica and Poisons *(pp. 53–61)*

1. Oliver David, Julian Clark, and Kytya Voeller, "Lead and Hyperactivity," *The Lancet*, October 28, 1972, pp. 900–903.
2. Mitchel W. Sauerhoff and J. Arthur Michaelson, "Hyperactivity and Brain Catecholamines in Lead-Exposed Developing Rats," *Science*, December 14, 1973, pp. 1022–1024.
3. Katherine Montague and Mercary Peter, *A Sierra Club Battlebook* (San Francisco, Sierra Club, 1971), pp. 15, 25, 33, 39, 51, 61, 71, 79, 93–94, 97–98.

Chapter 7.
Hyperactivity Caused by Brain Traumas *(pp. 62–65)*

1. Charles Bradley, M.D., "The Behavior of Children Receiving Benzedrine," *American Journal of Psychiatry*, November 1937, p. 578.
2. Evan W. Thomas, M.D., *Brain Injured Children with Special Reference to Doman-Delacato Methods of Treatment* (Springfield, Ill., Charles C. Thomas, 1969), pp. 54–60.

3. Dennis P. Cantwell, M.D., ed., et al., *The Hyperactive Child: Diagnosis, Management, Current Research* (New York, Spectrum Publications, 1976), p. 11.

Chapter 8.
Depression May Have a Physiological Base   (pp. 66–71)

1. Dennis P. Cantwell, M.D., ed., et al., *The Hyperactive Child: Diagnosis, Management, Current Research* (New York: Spectrum Publications, 1976), p. 180.
2. "G.W.," *Neuropsychiatric Bulletin*, Southern California Neuropsychiatric Institute, La Jolla, Ca. 92037, April–June, 1976, p. 1.

Chapter 9.
The "Myth" Makers   (pp. 75–79)

1. Nat Hentoff, "The Drugged Classroom," *Evergreen Review*, December 1970, as reproduced in *Current*, February 1971, pp. 40–45.
2. *Clinical Psychiatry News*, May 1976, pp. 3, 44.
3. Harlan Vinnedge, "Drugs for Children," *New Republic*, March 13, 1971, pp. 13–15.
4. Peter Schrag and Diane Divoky, *The Myth of the Hyperactive Child* (New York, Pantheon Books, 1975), pp. 35, 42.
5. Ibid., p. xvii.

Chapter 10.
What Ritalin Can and Can't Do   (pp. 80–92)

1. Maurice W. Laufer, M.D., *Journal of Learning Disabilities* 4, no. 9 (November 1971): 56–58.
2. Medicine Department, *Newsweek*, April 3, 1972.
3. Daniel Safer, M.D., Richard Allen, Ph.D., and Evelyn Barr, R.N., *New England Journal of Education*, August 3, 1972, pp. 217–220.
4. Gabrielle Weiss, M.D., et al., "Effects of Long-Term Treatment of Hyperactive Children with Methylphenidates," *Canadian Medical Association Journal*, January 25, 1975, pp. 159–165.
5. Domeena C. Renshaw, M.D., in the *Journal of the American Medical Association*, June 23, 1975, p. 1025.
6. Peggy Harmon, Bayside, N.Y., *Tourette Syndrome Association Newsletter* 4, no. 1 (January 1977).

Chapter 11.
Legal Drugs Can Be Dangerous   (pp. 93–100)

1. UPI, San Diego *Union*, August 16, 1976, p. K-2.
2. Charles Bradley, M.D., "The Behavior of Children Receiving Benzedrine," *American Journal of Psychiatry*, November 1937, pp. 577–585.
3. Charles Bradley, M.D., and Margaret Bowen, R.N., "Amphetamine (Benzedrine) Therapy of Children's Behavior Disorders," *American Journal of Orthopsychiatry*, November 1937, pp. 577–585; and Charles Bradley, M.D., "Benzedrine in the Treatment of Children's Behavior Disorders," *Pediatrics*, January 1950, pp. 24–26.
4. Nancy J. Cohen, Virginia I. Douglas, and Gert Morgenstern, "The Effect of Methylphenidate on Attentive Behavior and Autonomic Activity in Hyperactive Children," *Psychopharmacologia*, 1971, pp. 282–293.
5. Alexander R. Lucas, M.D., and Morris Weiss, M.D., "Methylphenidate Hallucinosis," *Journal of the American Medical Association*, August 23, 1971, pp. 1079–1081.
6. Mark A. Stewart, M.D. and Sally Wendkos Olds, *Raising a Hyperactive Child* (New York, Harper & Row, 1973).
7. Alan F. Charles, "The Case of Ritalin," *New Republic*, October 23, 1971, pp. 17–19.
8. HEW–OCD Report, *JLD* 4, no. 9 (November 1971): 63–65.
9. Dorothea M. Ross and Sheila A. Ross, *Hyperactivity: Research-Theory-Action* (New York, John Wiley, 1976), p. 113.
10. Gerald Solomons, M.D., "The Hyperkinetic Child," Medicine Department, *Newsweek*, April 3, 1972.
11. J. Claghorn, C. Neblett, E. Sutter, G. Farrell, and I. Kraft, "The Effect of Drugs on Hyperactivity in Children with Some Observations of Changes in Mineral Metabolism," *Journal of Nervous and Mental Disease* 153, no. 2, pp. 118–125.
12. L. Eugene Arnold, M.D., "The Art of Medicating Hyperkinetic Children," *Clinical Pediatrics*, January 1973, pp. 35–41.

Chapter 12.
Allergies and Hyperactivity   (pp. 101–106)

1. Doris J. Rapp, M.D., "Allergic-Tension-Fatigue Syndrome," *New Directions for Learning*, The New York Institute for Child Development, 205 Lexington Ave., New York, N.Y. 10016. This is one in a series of ongoing N.Y.I.C.D. projects.

2. Ben F. Feingold, M.D., *Why Your Child Is Hyperactive* (New York, Random House, 1975), p. 11.

3. "Teams Bid to Erase Allergies," San Diego *Union*, March 11, 1977, p. B-1. This is an ongoing research project at University of California San Diego Medical School, and may require five to ten years before completion.

Chapter 13.
Dr. Feingold's K-P Diet *(pp. 107–114)*

1. Ben F. Feingold, M.D., *Why Your Child Is Hyperactive*. (New York, Random House, 1975), pp. 13–14.

2. Ibid., p. 71.

3. Ibid., pp. 71–72.

4. Ibid., p. 72.

5. Ibid., pp. 30–43.

6. C. Christian Beels, "Economic Forces Challenge U.S. Economic Myth," San Diego *Union*, July 5, 1976, pp. D-1–D-2.

7. "Hyperkinesis: Does Subtracting Additives Help?" *Medical World News*, September 20, 1976, p. 50.

Chapter 14.
The "Patterning" Treatment *(pp. 115–122)*

1. Robert J. Doman, M.D., Eugene B. Spitz, M.D., Elizabeth Zucman, M.D., Carl H. Delacato, Ed.D., and Glenn Doman, P.T. (Dr. Doman and Dr. Zucman were identified as from the Rehabilitation Center at Philadelphia; Dr. Zucman, Ancien Externe des Hospitaux de Paris, was a research fellow during the course of this study; Dr. Spitz was from the Children's Hospital; and Delacato and G. Doman were also with the Rehabilitation Center), "Children with Severe Brain Injuries, Neurological Organization in Terms of Mobility," *Journal of the American Medical Association* 174, no. 3 (September 17, 1960): 257–262.

2. Ibid., p. 262.

3. Evan W. Thomas, M.D., *Brain-Injured Children with Special Reference to Doman-Delacato Methods of Treatment* (Springfield, Ill., Charles C. Thomas, 1969), introduction, pp. 15, 17, 74, 92.

4. Ibid., pp. 53–59.

5. Ibid., p. 124.

6. Ibid., pp. 105–115.

7. Virginia Apgar, M.D., M.P.H., and Joan Beck, *Is My Baby All Right?* (New York, Trident Press, 1972), p. 149.

8. Thomas, pp. 113–114.

Chapter 15.
Coffee   (pp. 123–126)

1. Robert C. Schnackenberg, M.D., "Caffeine as a Substitute for Schedule H Stimulants in Hyperkinetic Children," *American Journal of Psychiatry*, 130–7 (July 1973): 796–798.
2. *Psychiatric News*, August 6, 1975, p. 24.
3. Louis S. Goodman, M.D., and Alfred Gilman, M.D., *Pharmacological Basis of Therapeutics*, 3rd ed. (New York, Macmillan), Ch. 19.
4. "Coffee and Your Health," *Consumer Bulletin*, April 1971, p. 22.

Chapter 16.
Megavitamins   (pp. 127–134)

1. HEW-OCD Report, reprinted in *Journal of Learning Diasabilities* 4, no. 9 (November 1971): 65–66.
2. Sydney Walker, III, M.D., *Psychiatric Signs and Symptoms Due to Medical Problems* (Springfield, Ill., Charles C. Thomas, 1967), pp. 178–179.
3. Ibid., pp. 179–180.
4. Robert J. Trotter, "Will Vitamins Replace the Psychiatrist's Couch?" *Science News* 104 (July 28, 1973): 59–60.
5. San Diego *Evening Tribune*, December 14, 1976, p. B-1; San Diego *Union*, December 16, 1976, p. D-1.

Chapter 17.
Lithium   (pp. 135–139)

1. *Lithium in the Treatment of Mood Disorders*, National Institute of Mental Health, National Clearinghouse for Mental Health Information, Pub. No. 5033 (1970), pp. 13–14.
2. Ibid., pp. 31–35.
3. Ibid., p. 67.
4. Ibid., p. 66.
5. W. Clifford M. Scott, letter, *British Medical Journal*, April 14, 1973, pp. 113–114.
6. *Lithium*, p. 63.
7. Ibid., p. 68.
8. Lawrence L. Greenhill, M.D., Ronald O. Rieder, M.D., Paul H. Wender, M.D., Monte Buchsbaum, M.D., Theodore P. Zahn, Ph.D., "Lithium Carbonate in the Treatment of Hyperactive Chil-

dren," *Arch Gen Psychiatry* 28, May 1973, pp. 636–640.
9. *Lithium*, pp. 22–24.

Chapter 18.
Brain Surgery: The Irreversible Treatment   (pp. 140–143)

1. H. Krayenbuhl, and J. Siegfried, "Dentatomies or Thalamotomies in the Treatment of Hyperkinesia," *Confinia Neurologica* 34 (1972): 29–33.
2. Phyllis Breggin, "Is Psychosurgery an Acceptable Treatment of Hyperactivity in Children?" *Mental Hygiene*, Winter 1974, pp. 19–21.
3. Ibid., p. 20.

Chapter 20.
When a Psychiatrist Is Needed   (pp. 165–169)

1. Jerry Newton, M.D. (School Health Services, San Antonio, Texas), "Minimal Brain Dysfunction: Towards an Understanding Between School and Physician," *Journal of the American Medical Association*, June 7, 1976, pp. 2524–2525.
2. International Medical News Service, "Psychiatrists Losing Image of Being M.D.," *Clinical Psychiatry News*, July 1976, p. 1.
3. International Medical News Service, "It Is Time Psychiatrists Stopped Avoiding Laying On of Hands," *Clinical Psychiatry News*, July 1976, p. 1.
4. "S.W. III and G.W.," editorial, *Neuropsychiatric Bulletin*, First Quarter, 1976, Southern California Neuropsychiatric Institute, La Jolla, California.

Chapter 22.
Parents' Resources and the Future   (pp. 184–191)

1. In *Reaching Children*, Operation Learning Bulletin, published by the New York Institute for Child Development, 205 Lexington Ave., New York, N.Y. 10016.

Index